2017 G
Buyers Guide

© 2017 The Gluten Free Buyers Guide is a guide to achieving better health for those with Gluten Intolerance and or Celiac Disease. It is written with your needs in mind but is not a substitute for consulting with your physician or other health care providers. The publisher and authors are not responsible for any adverse effects or consequences resulting from the use of the suggestions, products or procedures that appear in this guide. Any product claim, statistic, quote or other representation about a product, service, or organization should be verified with the manufacturer or provider. All matters regarding your health should be supervised by a licensed health care physician.

Copyright © 2014 - 2017 by Jayme Schieffer and Josh Schieffer, The Gluten Free Buyers Guide.com All rights reserved.

Table of Contents

Introduction by Josh Schieffer 6
Bagels 8
Beer Brands 10
Blogs 12
Books 16
Bread Brands 20
Bread Crumbs 22
Bread Mixes 24
Breakfast On-The-Go 26
Brownie Mix 28
Cake Mix 30
Children's Book 32
Cold Cereal 34
Colleges for Gluten-Free Students 36
Comfort Food 38
Cookbooks 40
Cookie Mixes 44
Cookies 46
Cornbread Mix 48
Cosmetic Brands 50
Crackers 52
Donuts 56
Expo and Events 57
Flours 58

Frozen Meals.. 60
Frozen Pancake & Waffle Brands............................ 62
Frozen Pizza Brands... 64
Granola.. 66
Jerky 68
Magazines 70
Mobile Apps 72
Muffin Mix.. 74
Munchies.. 76
National Restaurant Chains 78
New Products... 80
Non-Profits.. 82
Online Resources 84
Online Stores.. 86
Pancake and Waffle Mixes 88
Pastas 90
Pie Crust 92
Pizza Crust Mix 94
Ready Made Desserts 96
Sauces... 98
Shopping Guide... 100
Snack Bars... 102
Social Media Platforms 104
Summer Camps 106
Supplements... 108
Tortilla or Wrap 110

2017 Gluten Free Buyers Guide

Vacation Destinations 112
Website 114

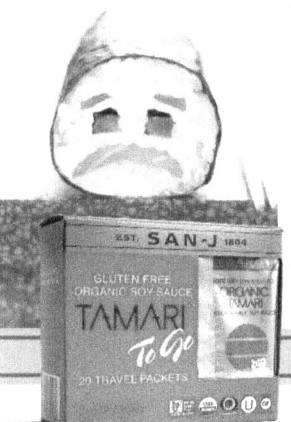

Your takeout has been lonely too long.

Gluten-free is now hassle-free.

Is that restaurant or take out soy sauce gluten-free? Usually no — and often, there's no way to tell. But now with San-J's convenient Tamari To Go travel packs, it's easy to bring your favorite gluten-free taste with you anytime! Eating in or taking out — for sushi, tofu, fresh spring rolls, or as a delicious alternative to salt — you never need to be without the rich gourmet flavor of San-J's famous organic Tamari soy sauce!

EST. **SAN-J** 1804

©2014 San-J International, Inc. www.san-j.com

Introduction by Josh Schieffer

First of all, let me thank you for picking up this book. We are delighted you have decided to find the best in gluten-free. This book has been carefully designed to help you quickly connect with the best gluten-free products, services, and organizations. We host the Annual Gluten-Free Awards; a program that enables the gluten-free community to cast votes for their favorites. This year we had 3527 people take part in the voting process. The 96,128 individual responses are all rolled up in the following pages.

This year we added a few new award categories now totaling 51.

About us

Initially we started the awards program with a one page website in 2010 with just a few categories. At that time and even now, there is no single source to find the best gluten-free products in multiple categories.

Families, including us, would struggle financially while experimenting with terrible tasting gluten-free products during the transition process. Fast forward a few years and we are now reaching hundreds of thousands of people, industry leaders, and most importantly YOU. We continue to grow each year with new categories and resources based on community feedback.

We want to make sure you truly understand what is gluten free or not. For years, we have excluded gluten removed beers and other conservational products. Some people want certified gluten free products listen while others want to see a gluten free listed ingredients list. Here's the bottom line, we try our best to make sure our family including yours has the best gluten free products. Please ensure producers of these listed gluten free products have not changed their ingredient listings and or their gluten free certifications.

Please reach out to us at Gluten Free Buyers Guide.com if you have any questions or want to give us some feedback.

Again, we do this for you.

Bagels

7th Annual Gluten-Free Awards:
1st Place: Canyon Bakehouse Plain Bagels

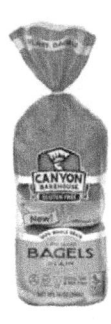

2nd Place: Canyon Bakehouse Everything Bagels

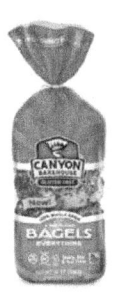

3rd Place: BFree Multiseed Bagel

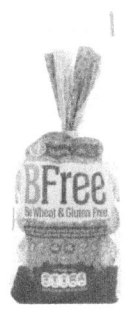

2017 Gluten Free Buyers Guide

Other Nominees:

BFree White Bagel

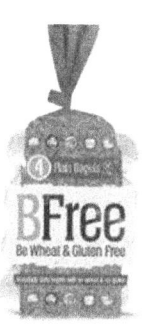

Sweet Note Bakery Everything Bagels

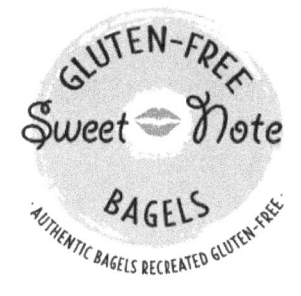

Sweet Note Bakery Plain Bagels

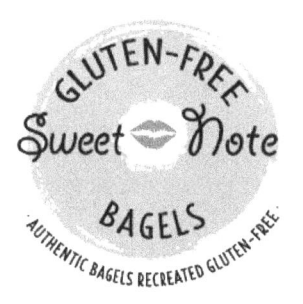

Beer Brands

7th Annual Gluten-Free Awards:
1st Place: Redbridge

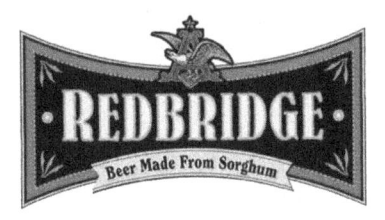

2nd Place: Glutenberg

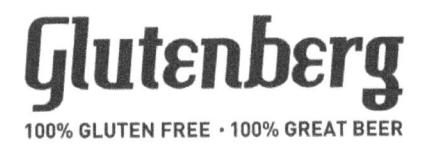

3rd Place: New Planet

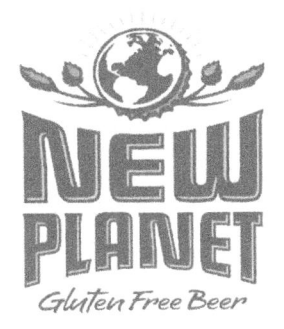

Other Nominees:

Green's

2017 Gluten Free Buyers Guide

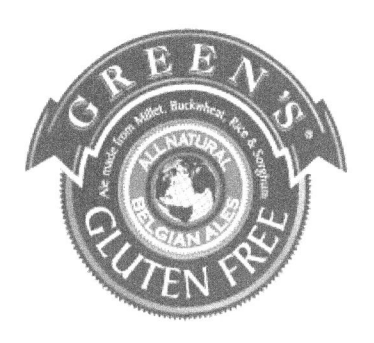

Bards

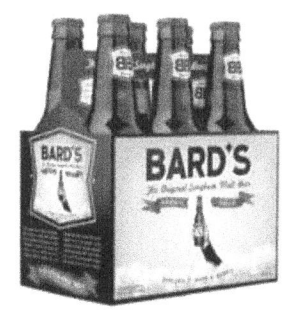

Ground Breaker Brewing

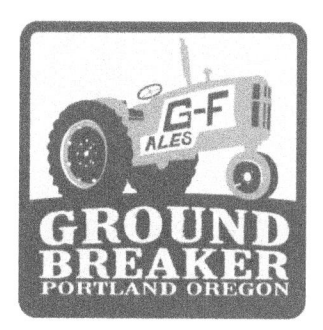

St. Peter's

Celia Saison

Blogs

7th Annual Gluten-Free Awards:
1st Place: GF Jules

http://gfjules.com/

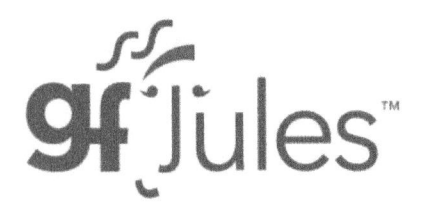

2nd Place: Gluten-Free on a Shoestring
http://glutenfreeonashoestring.com/

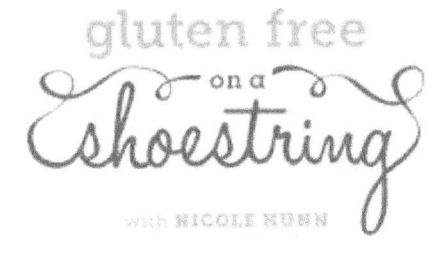

3rd Place: Gluten Dude

http://glutendude.com/

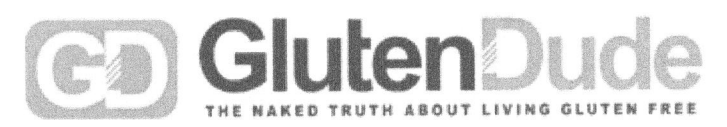

Other nominees:

Gluten Free Girl

https://glutenfreegirl.com/

Celiac and the Beast

http://celiacandthebeast.com/

What The Fork Food Blog

http://www.whattheforkfoodblog.com/

Rasing Jack with Celiac

http://www.raisingjackwithceliac.com/

My Gluten Free Kitchen

http://mygluten-freekitchen.com/

Gluten Free & Dairy Free at WDW

Http://www.glutenfreedairyfreewdw.com/

Gluten Free & More

http://www.glutenfreeandmore.com/

Vegetarian Mamma

http://vegetarianmamma.com/

Jennifer's Way

http://jennifersway.org/myblog/

Yum Food for Living

http://yumfoodforliving.com/

Tasty Meditation

https://tastymeditation.wordpress.com/

Gluten Free Easily

http://glutenfreeeasily.com/

Celtic Celiac

http://www.celticceliac.com/

GF Mom Certified

http://vphonegirl.blogspot.com/

Flippin Delicious

http://flippindelicious.com/

Gluten-Free Globetrotter

https://glutenfreeglobetrotter.com/

Gluten Free Follow Me

http://www.glutenfreefollowme.com/

All Day I Dream About Food

http://alldayidreamaboutfood.com/

Love G Free Life

https://lovegfreelife.wordpress.com/

Unconventional Baker

http://www.unconventionalbaker.com/

I'm a Celiac

http://www.imaceliac.com/

Gluten Free Makeovers

http://glutenfreemakeovers.com/

Gluten Away

http://glutenaway.blogspot.com/

Alexis Gluten Free Adventures

http://www.gfinorlando.com/

Gluten Free Palate

http://www.glutenfreepalate.com/

Only Taste Matters

http://onlytastematters.com/

King Gluten Free

http://www.kingglutenfree.com/

Free Range Cookies

http://freerangecookies.com/

The Adventures of Anti-Wheat Girl

http://antiwheatgirl.com/

Agony Of De Wheat

http://www.agonyofdewheat.com/

Grain Changer

http://grainchanger.com/

Strength and Sunshine

http://strengthandsunshine.com/

CAFE by Jackie Ourman

http://jackieourman.com/

Dishes for Libby

http://dishesforlibby.com/

NoBread

http://nobread.com/about

Beard and Bonnet

http://beardandbonnet.com/

Books

7th Annual Gluten-Free Awards:

1st Place: The First Year: Celiac Disease and Living Gluten-Free: An Essential Guide for the Newly Diagnosed: Jules Shepard

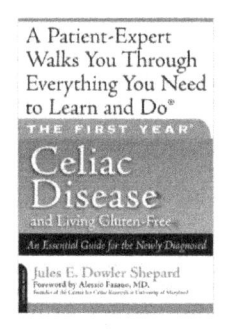

2nd Place: Jennifer's Way: My Journey with Celiac Disease--What Doctors Don't Tell You and How You Can Learn to Live Again by Jennifer Esposito

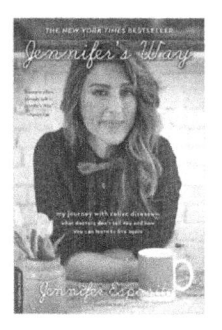

3rd Place: Celiac and the Beast: A Love Story Between a Gluten-Free Girl, Her Genes, and a Broken Digestive Tract by Erica Dermer

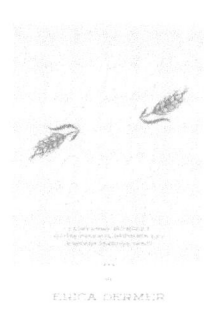

Other Nominees:

Gluten Freedom: The Nation's Leading Expert Offers the Essential Guide to a Healthy, Gluten-Free Lifestyle by Alessio Fasano (Author), Susie Flaherty (Contributor)

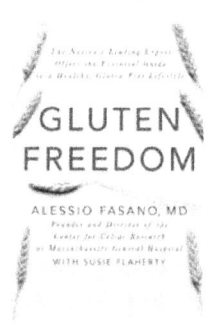

Kid Approved Mom Certified: Tiffany Hinton

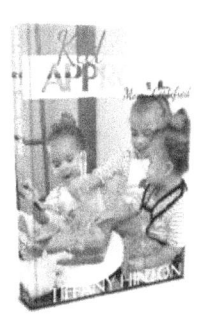

The Gluten Free Revolution: Jax Peters Lowell

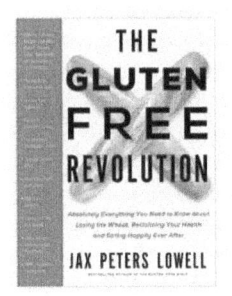

2017 Gluten Free Buyers Guide — 19

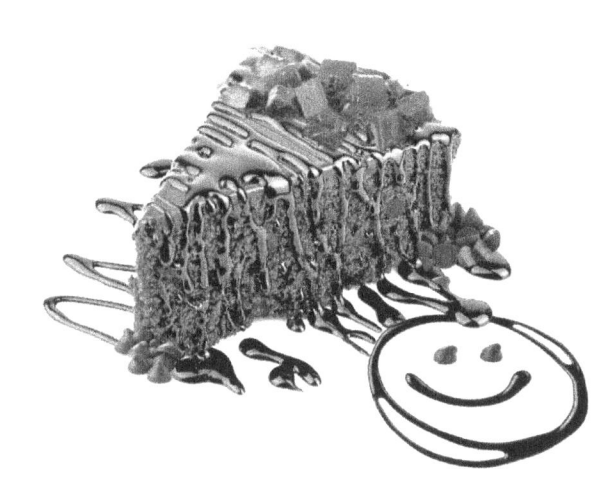

PURE DELIGHT
NO SOY · NO DAIRY · ALL CHOCOLATE

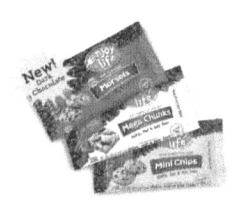

Make the deliciously sweet and safe choice with Enjoy Life **Semi-Sweet Mini Chips, Mega Chunks** and NEW **Dark Morsels**! They're dairy and nut free as well as free from the 8 most common allergens, and because we don't use soy fillers, there's room for more pure chocolate! All our chocolate is created in a dedicated nut free facility, so you can eat freely while enjoying every bit of chocolate decadence.

EAT FREELY, ENJOY FULLY

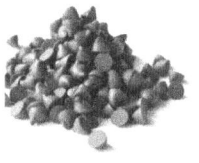

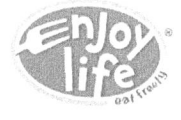

enjoylifefoods.com   #eatfreely

Enjoy Life — eat freely

Bread Brands

7th Annual Gluten-Free Awards:

1st Place: Canyon Bakehouse 7-Grain Bread

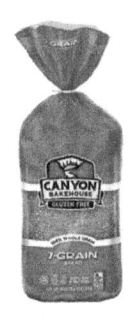

2nd Place: Canyon Bakehouse Mountain White Bread

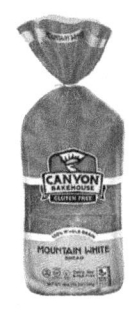

3rd Place: Schär Artisan Baker White Bread

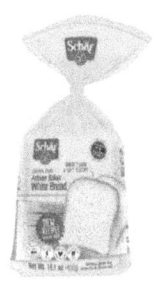

Other nominees:

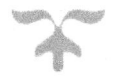

2017 Gluten Free Buyers Guide

Udi's Gluten Free Whole Grain Bread

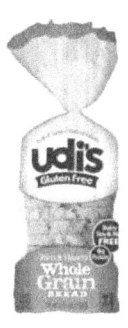

Schär Artisan Baker Multi-grain Bread

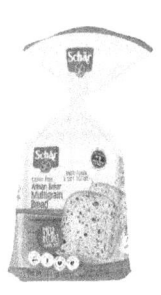

Aldi's LiveGfree Gluten Free Whole Grain Bread

Udi's Gluten Free White Bread

BFree Brown Seeded Loaf

BFree White Loaf

La Brea Bakery Gluten-Free Multigrain Artisan Sliced Sandwich Bread

La Brea Bakery Gluten-Free White Artisan Sliced Sandwich Bread

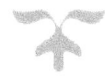

Bread Crumbs

7th Annual Gluten-Free Awards:
1st Placer: Schar Gluten Free Bread Crumbs

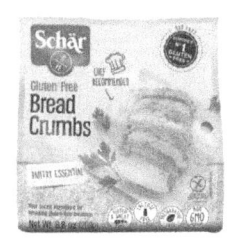

2nd Place: Ian's Italian Panko Breadcrumbs Ian's

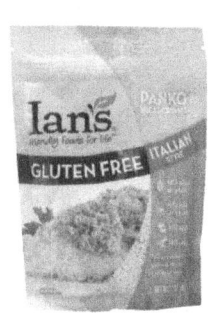

3rd Place: 4C Gluten Free Seasoned Crumbs

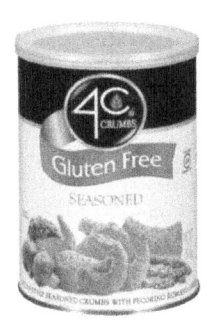

Other nominees:

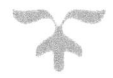

2017 Gluten Free Buyers Guide

Aleia's Gluten Free Panko Crumbs

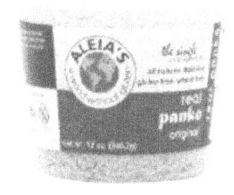

Gillian's Foods Bread Crumbs Gluten Free Italian

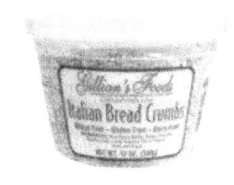

Tall Papa Gluten-Free Italian Seasoned Multi-Grain Bread Crumbs

Bread Mixes

7th Annual Gluten-Free Awards:
1st Place: gfJules Bread Mix

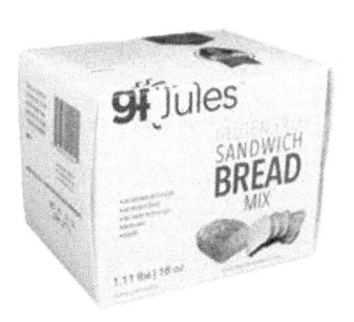

2nd Place: Aldi's liveGfree Gluten Free Cornbread Mix

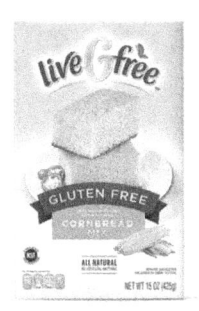

3rd Place: Enjoy Life All-Purpose Flour

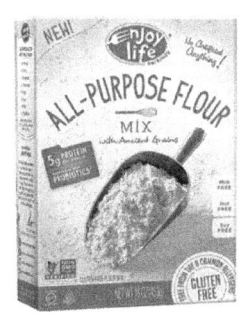

Other nominees:

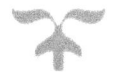

Namaste Bread & Roll Mix

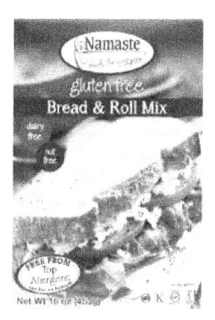

Aldi's liveGfree Gluten Free Pizza Crust Mix

Breads From Anna Banana Bread Mix

Stone Wall Kitchen Gluten Free Cornbread Mix

Luce's Gluten-Free Artisan Bread

Blackbird Bakes Bread & Pizza Blend

Mehl's Flour Mix

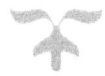

Breakfast On-The-Go

7th Annual Gluten-Free Awards:
1st Place: Canyon Oats Gluten Free Maple Oatmeal

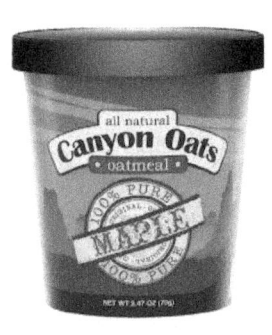

2nd Place: Luna Protein Chocolate Chip Cookie

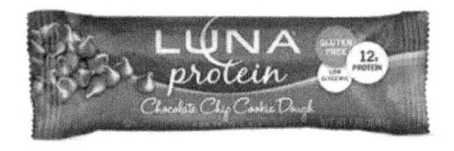

3rd Place: Enjoy Life Fruit & Seed Mix

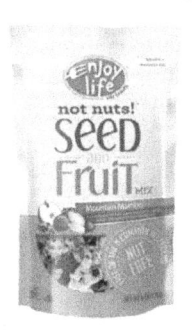

Other nominees:

2017 Gluten Free Buyers Guide

Enjoy Life Sunseed Crunch Bars

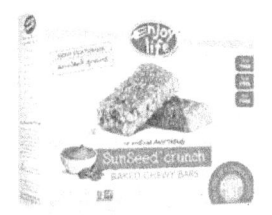

Mikey's Muffins Original English Muffin

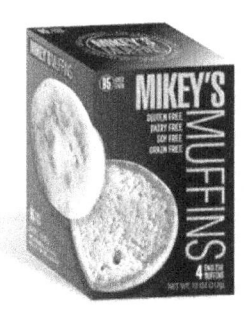

Oatmega Bars

Freedom Foods TropicO's

Brownie Mix

7th Annual Gluten-Free Awards:
1st Place: gfJules Brownie Mix

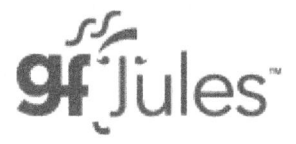

2nd Place: King Arthur Flour Gluten Free Brownie Mix

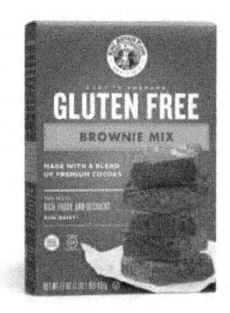

3rd Place: Trader Joe's Gluten Free Brownie Mix

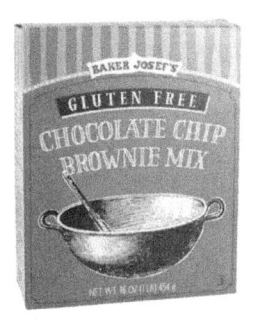

Other Nominees:

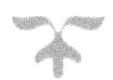

2017 Gluten Free Buyers Guide

Enjoy Life Brownie Mix

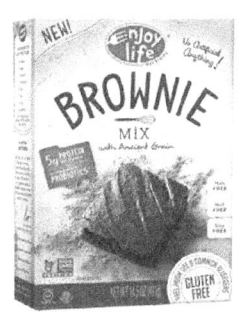

Hannah's Healthy Paleo Brownie Mix

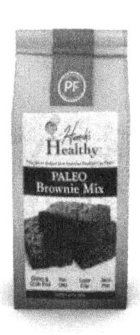

Cake Mix

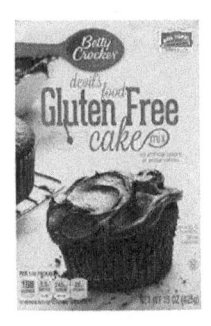

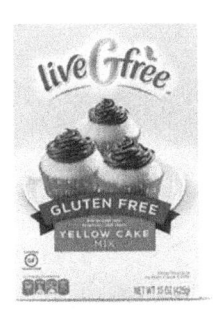

7th Annual Gluten-Free Awards:
1st Place: Betty Crocker Gluten Free Chocolate Cake Mix

2nd Place: Aldi's LiveGfree Gluten Free Yellow Cake Mix

2017 Gluten Free Buyers Guide

3rd Place: My Grandpa's Farm Organic Pumpkin Spice Gluten Free Cake Mix

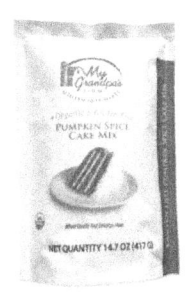

Other Nominees:

Abundant Love Premium Gluten Free Cake Mix

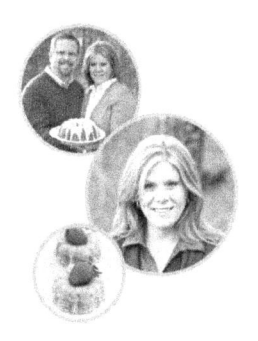

Children's Book

7th Annual Gluten-Free Awards:

1st Place: Eat Like a Dinosaur: Recipe & Guidebook for Gluten-free Kids by Paleo Parents and Elana Amsterdam

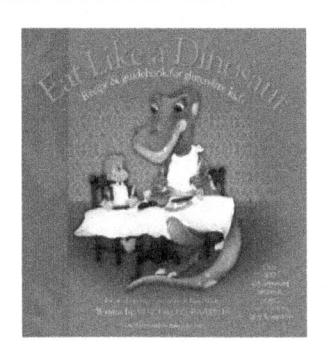

2nd Place: The GF Kid: A Celiac Disease Survival Guide by Melissa London and Eric Glickman

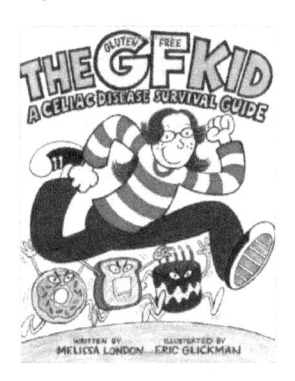

3rd Place: Kid Approved: Mom Certified by Tiffany Hinton

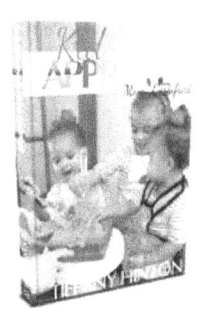

Other nominees:

Eating Gluten-Free with Emily: A Story for Children with Celiac Disease by Bonnie J. Kruszka and Richard S. Cihlar

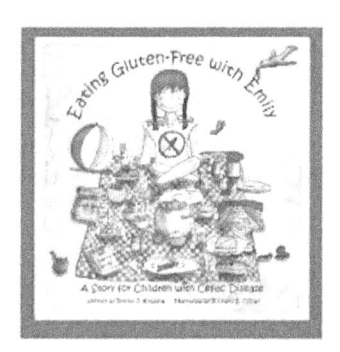

Adam's Gluten Free Surprise: Helping Others Understand Gluten Free by Debbie Simpson

Gordy and the Magic Diet by by Kim Diersen (Author), April Runge (Author), Carrie Hartman (Illustrator)

The Gluten Glitch by Stasie John and Kevin Cannon

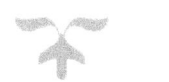

Cold Cereal

7th Annual Gluten-Free Awards:
1st Place: General Mills Cinnamon Chex

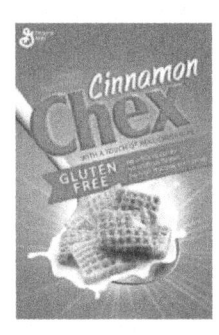

2nd Place: Gluten Free Honey Nut Cheerios

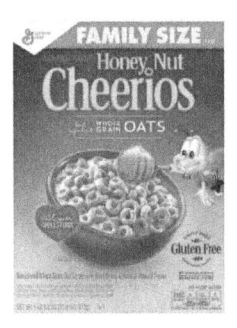

3rd Place: Envirokids Panda Puffs

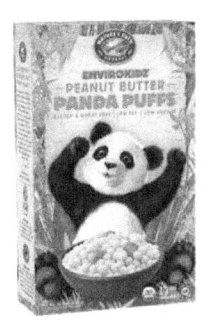

Other nominees:

2017 Gluten Free Buyers Guide

Nature's Path Mesa Sunrise

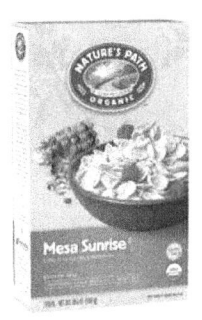

Gluten Free Special K

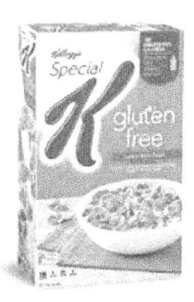

Bakery On Main's Bunches of Crunches

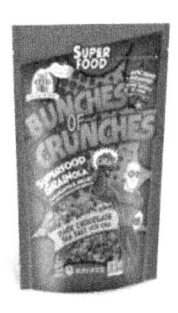

Back To Nature Gluten-Free Sprouted Whole Grain Brown Rice Crisps "Sprout and Shine"

Freedom Foods Tropico's

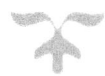

Colleges for Gluten-Free Students

7th Annual Gluten-Free Awards:

1st Place: KENT STATE UNIVERSITY

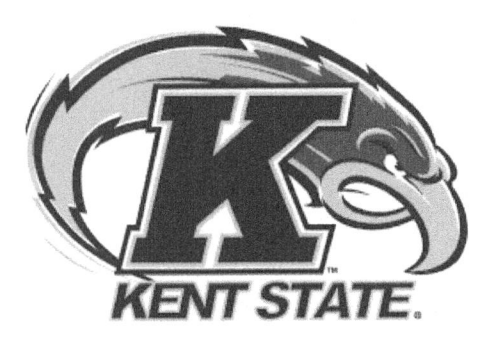

2nd Place: UNIVERSITY OF COLORADO: BOULDER

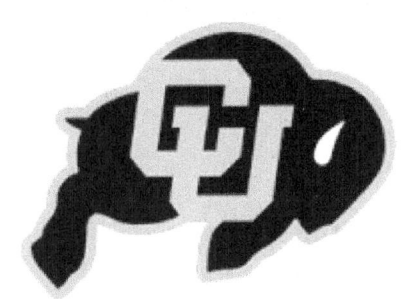

3rd Place: UNIVERSITY OF NOTRE DAME

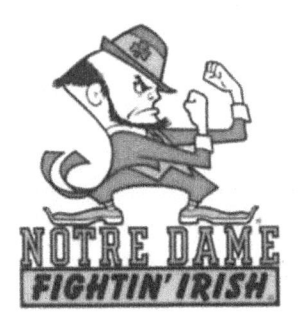

Other nominees:

NC STATE UNIVERSITY

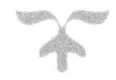

UNIVERSITY OF TENNESSEE

UNIVERSITY OF ARIZONA

SAN DIEGO STATE

OREGON STATE UNIVERSITY

YALE UNIVERSITY

IOWA STATE UNIVERSITY

UNIVERSITY OF CONNECTICUT

ITHACA COLLEGE

UNIVERSITY OF NEW HAMPSHIRE

GEORGETOWN UNIVERSITY

COLUMBIA UNIVERSITY

TOWSON UNIVERSITY

CLARK UNIVERSITY

CARLETON COLLEGE

Comfort Food

7th Annual Gluten-Free Awards:
1st Place: Annie's Mac and Cheese

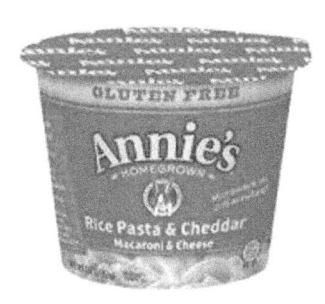

2nd Place: Amy's Mac n Cheese

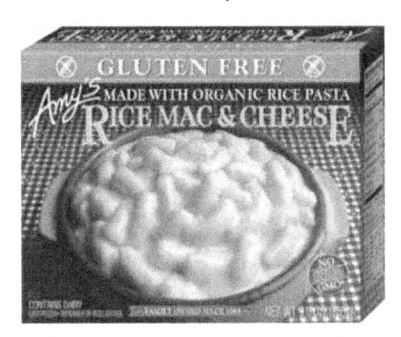

3rd Place: Progresso Gluten Free New England Clam Chowder

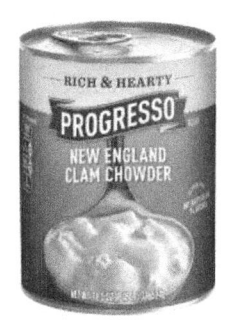

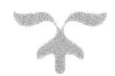

Other nominees:

2017 Gluten Free Buyers Guide

Gluten Free Territory Raspberry Brownies

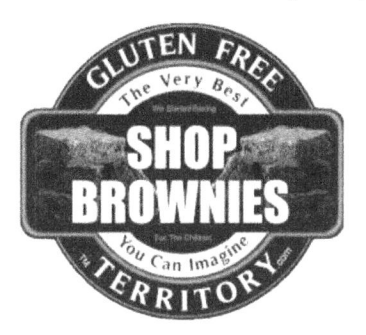

San-J White Miso Soup

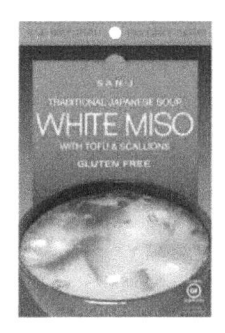

Cookbooks

7th Annual Gluten-Free Awards:

1st Place: Gluten-Free on a Shoestring, Quick and Easy: 100 Recipes for the Food You Love--Fast! by Nicole Hunn

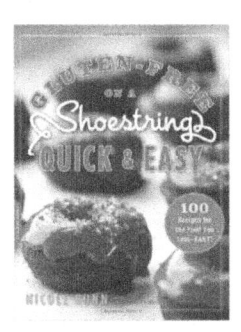

2nd Place: Free for All Cooking: 150 Easy Gluten-Free, Allergy-Friendly Recipes the Whole Family Can Enjoy by Jules E. Dowler Shepard

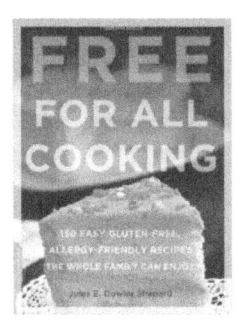

3rd Place: The How Can It Be Gluten Free Cookbook Paperback by America's Test Kitchen (Editor)

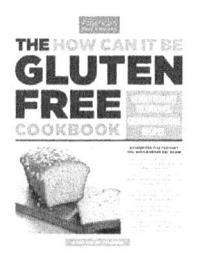

Other nominees:

Gluten-Free Quick & Easy: From Prep to Plate Without the Fuss - 200+ Recipes for People with Food Sensitivities by Carol Fenster Ph.D.

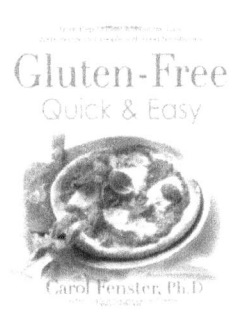

The Lagasse Girls' Big Flavor, Bold Taste--and No Gluten!: 100 Gluten-Free Recipes from EJ's Fried Chicken to Momma's Strawberry Shortcake by Jilly Lagasse and Jessie Lagasse Swanson

Artisanal Gluten-Free Cooking: 275 Great-Tasting, From-Scratch Recipes from Around the World,

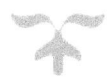

Perfect for Every Meal and for Anyone on a Gluten-Free Dietand Even Those Who Aren't Paperback by Kelli Bronski and Peter Bronski

Paleo Takeout: Restaurant Favorites Without the Junk Paperback by Russ Crandall

YUM: plant-based recipes for a gluten-free diet by Theresa Nicassio

Sweet & Simple Gluten-Free Baking: Irresistible Classics in 10 Ingredients or Less! by Chrystal Carver

The Everyday Art of Gluten-Free: 125 Savory and Sweet Recipes Using 6 Fail-Proof Flour Blends by Karen Morgan

Mom Certified Celebrates Heritage by Tiffany Hinton

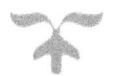

2017 Gluten Free Buyers Guide

· DAIRY FREE · TREE NUT FREE · GMO FREE · **FREE FROM** · EGG FREE · GLUTEN FREE · WHEAT FREE ·

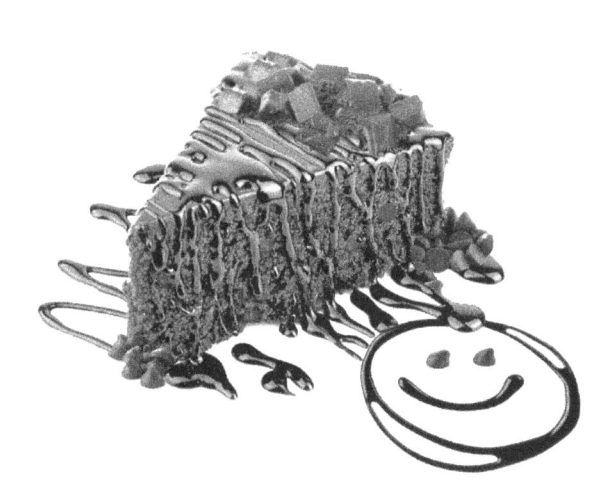

PURE DELIGHT
NO SOY · NO DAIRY · ALL CHOCOLATE

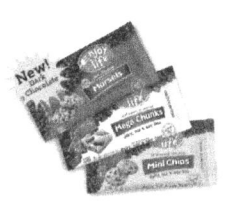

Make the deliciously sweet and safe choice with Enjoy Life Semi-Sweet Mini Chips, Mega Chunks and NEW Dark Morsels! They're dairy and nut free as well as free from the 8 most common allergens, and because we don't use soy fillers, there's room for more pure chocolate! All our chocolate is created in a dedicated nut free facility, so you can eat freely while enjoying every bit of chocolate decadence.

EAT FREELY, ENJOY FULLY

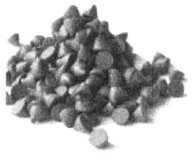

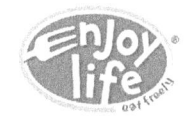

Learn more about our complete line of delicious Free From products at
enjoylifefoods.com   #eatfreely

enjoy life
eat freely

· PEANUT FREE · DAIRY FREE · EGG FREE · FREE FROM · GMO FREE · TREE NUT FREE · SOY FREE ·

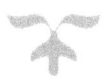

Cookie Mixes

7th Annual Gluten-Free Awards:
1st Place: gfJules Original Cookie Mix

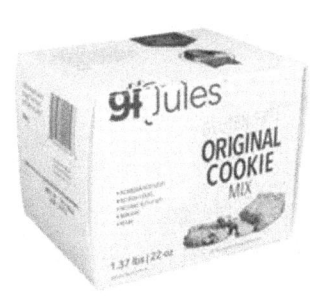

2nd Place: Betty Crocker Gluten-Free Chocolate Chip Mix

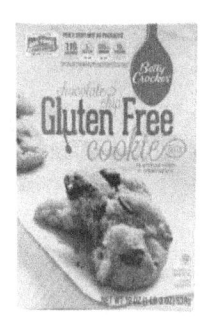

3rd Place Pamela's Chocolate Chip Cookie Mix

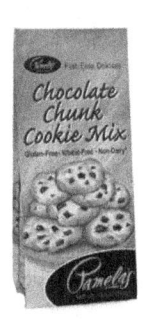

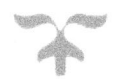

Other nominees:

2017 Gluten Free Buyers Guide

Namaste Cookie Mix

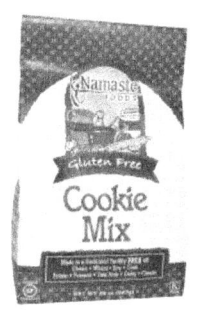

Stonewall Kitchen Gluten Free Chocolate Chip Cookie Mix

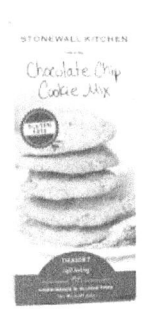

Among Friends Suzie Q's Oatmeal Chocolate Chip Cookie Mix

Eat Pastry Gluten-Free Sugar Momma Cookie Dough

Blackbird Bakes Cookie Jar Mix

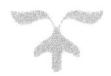

Cookies

7th Annual Gluten-Free Awards:

1st Place: Tate's Chocolate Chip

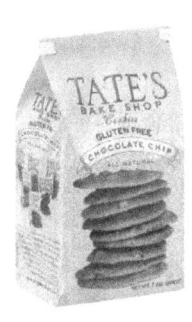

2nd Place: Glutino Lemon Wafers

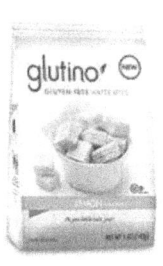

3rd Place: Enjoy Life's Double Chocolate Brownie Soft Baked Cookies

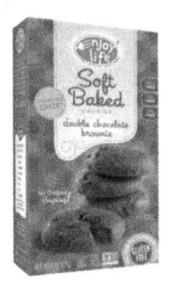

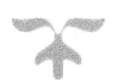

Other nominees:

2017 Gluten Free Buyers Guide

Enjoy Life's Snickerdoodle Mini Cookies

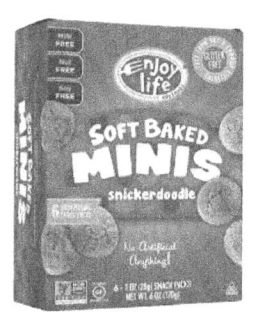

Glutino Animal Cracker- Graham

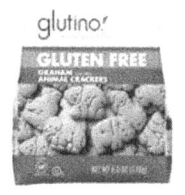

Lucy's Maple Bliss

Aleia's Chocolate Chip Cookie Gluten Free

ginnybakes Chocolate Chip Macadamia Cookie Love

Nairn's Gluten-Free Original Oat Grahams

Nairn's Gluten-Free Chocolate Chip Oat Grahams

Cornbread Mix

7th Annual Gluten-Free Awards:
1st Place: gfJules Cornbread Mix

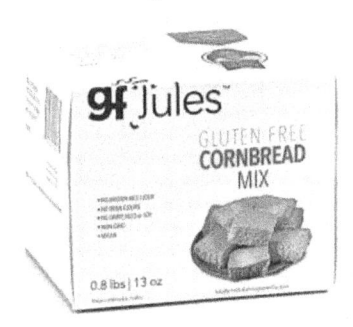

2nd Place: Krusteaz Gluten Free Honey Cornbread Mix

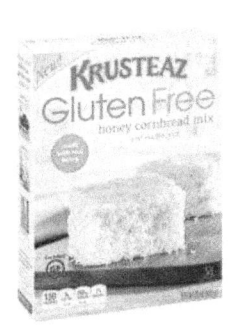

3rd Place: Aldi's LiveGfree Gluten Free Cornbread Mix

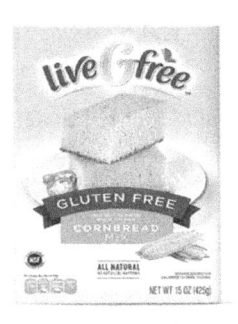

2017 Gluten Free Buyers Guide   49

Other nominees:

Gluten Free Bakehouse Cornbread

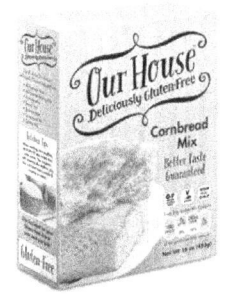

Cosmetic Brands

7th Annual Gluten-Free Awards:
1st Place: tarte

tarte
high-performance naturals™

2nd Place: Arbonne

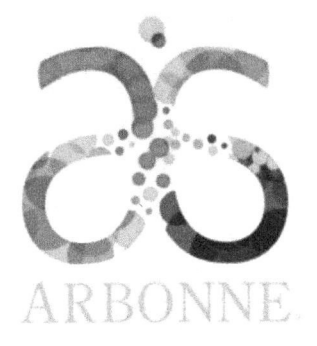

ARBONNE

3rd Place: Red Apple Lipstick

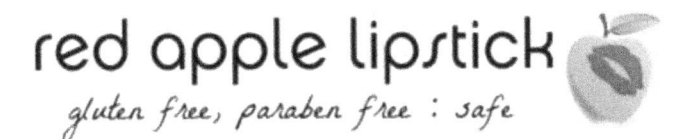

red apple lipstick
gluten free, paraben free : safe

Other nominees:

Mineral Fusion

100% Pure

Juice Beauty

Ecco Bella

Afterglow

Acure

Au Naturale

Vbeauté

Crackers

7th Annual Gluten-Free Awards:
1st Place: Schär Table Crackers

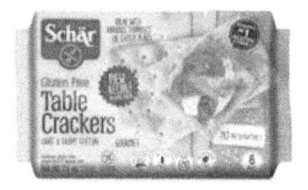

2nd Place: Crunchmaster Original

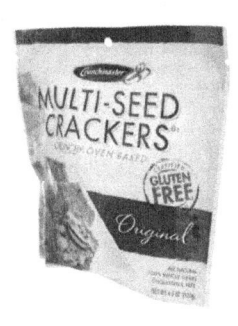

3rd Place: Aldi's LiveGfree Gluten Free Rosemary & Olive Oil Multiseed Crackers

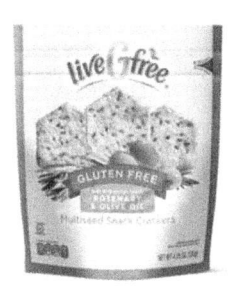

Other nominees:

2017 Gluten Free Buyers Guide   53

Van's Say Cheese! Crackers

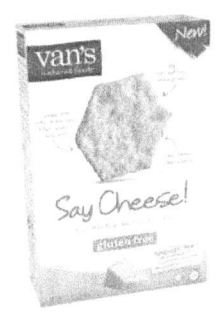

Mary's Gone Crackers: Original

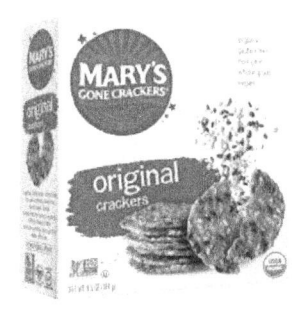

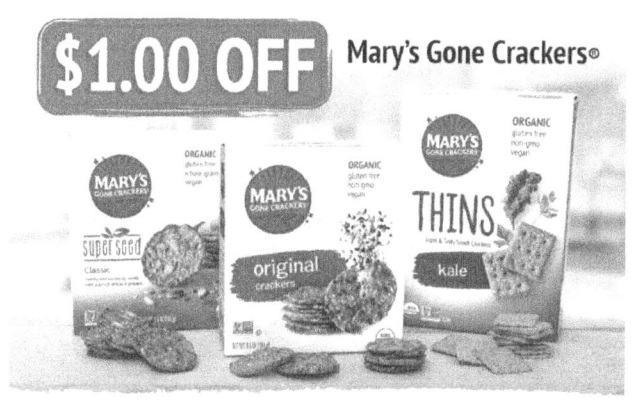

$1.00 OFF Mary's Gone Crackers®

$1.00 OFF ANY MGC PRODUCT

MANUFACTURER'S COUPON | EXPIRES 12/31/17

0897580000-130080

RETAILER: MARY'S GONE CRACKERS® will reimburse you the face value of this coupon plus 8¢ handling provided it is redeemed by a consumer at the time of purchase on the brand specified. Coupons not properly redeemed will be void and held. Reproduction of this coupon is expressly prohibited. (Any other use constitutes fraud.) Mail to: INMAR Dep't 97580, Mary's Gone Crackers, 1 Fawcett Drive, Del Rio, TX 78840. Cash value .001¢. Void where taxed or restricted. Limit one coupon per item purchased.

CONSCIOUS EATING
For the health of body, mind and planet™.
www.marysgonecrackers.com

2017 Gluten-Free Buyers Guide

Simple Mills Farmhouse Cheddar

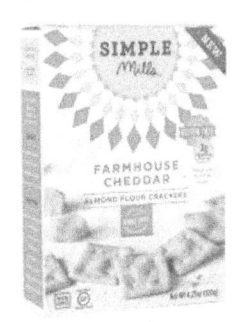

San-J Tamari Black Sesame Crackers

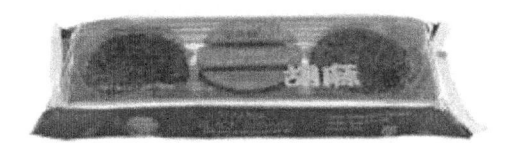

Saffron Road Sea Salt Lentil Crackers

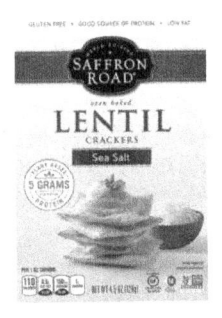

2017 Gluten Free Buyers Guide

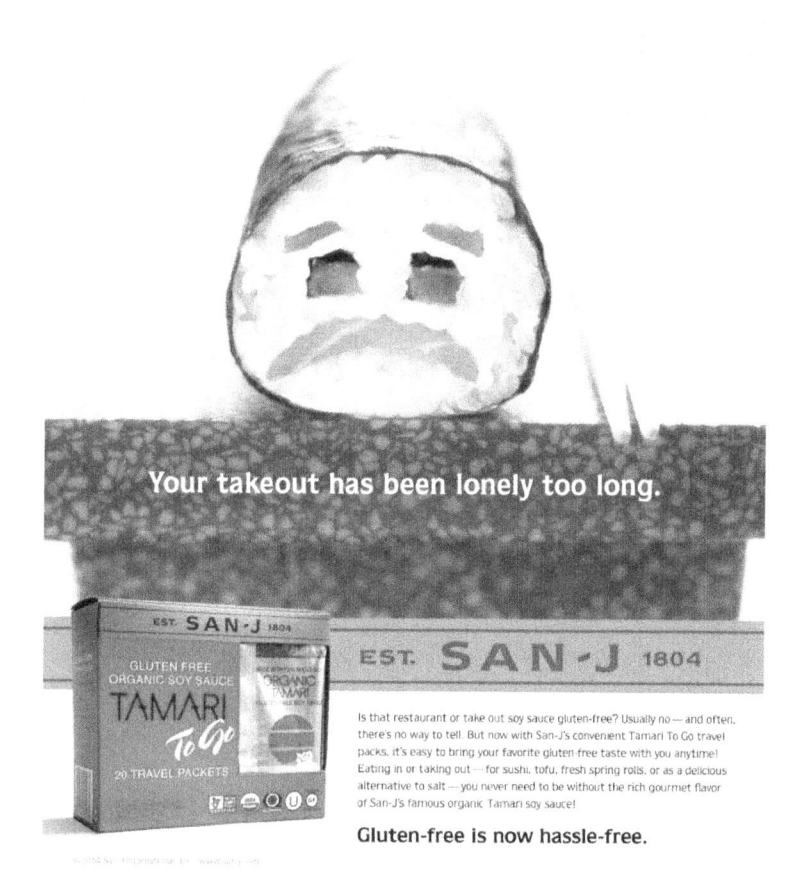

Your takeout has been lonely too long.

EST. SAN-J 1804

Is that restaurant or take out soy sauce gluten-free? Usually no — and often, there's no way to tell. But now with San-J's convenient Tamari To Go travel packs, it's easy to bring your favorite gluten free taste with you anytime! Eating in or taking out — for sushi, tofu, fresh spring rolls, or as a delicious alternative to salt — you never need to be without the rich gourmet flavor of San-J's famous organic Tamari soy sauce!

Gluten-free is now hassle-free.

Donuts
7th Annual Gluten-Free Awards:
1st Place: Kinnikinnick Donuts

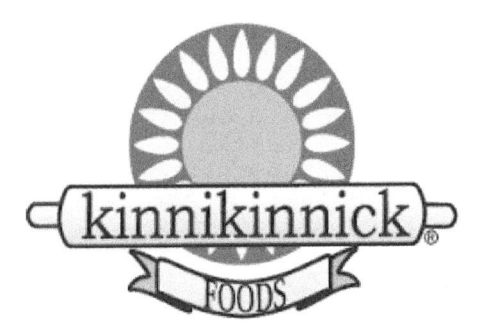

2nd Place: Katz

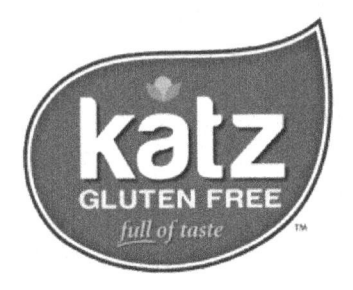

3rd Place: Bare Naked Bakery Donuts

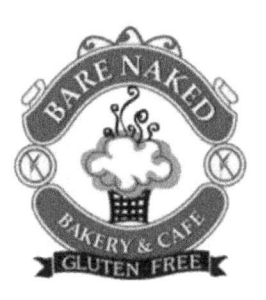

Expo and Events

7th Annual Gluten-Free Awards:

1st Place: Gluten & Allergen Free Expos

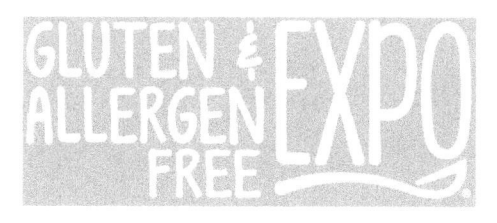

2nd Place: Living Without's Gluten Free Food Allergy Fest

3rd Place: The GlutenAway Online Expo

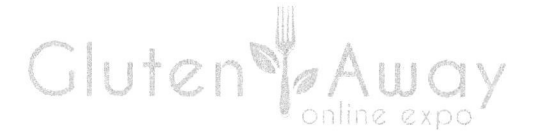

Other nominees:

Gluten & Allergen Free Wellness Events

Natural Products Expo West / East

CDF National Education & Gluten-Free Expo

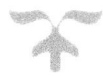

Flours

7th Annual Gluten-Free Awards:

1st Place: gfJules Gluten Free All Purpose Flour

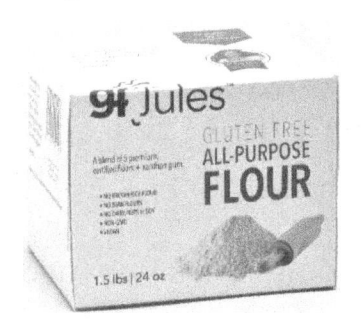

2nd Place: Bob's Red Mill 1-to-1

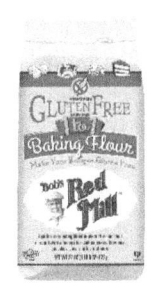

3rd Place: King Arthur Flour Multi-Purpose

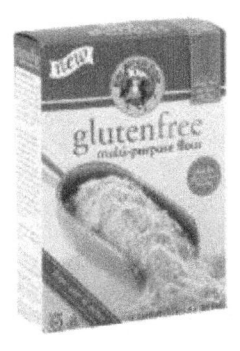

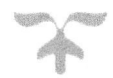

Other nominees:

2017 Gluten Free Buyers Guide

Cup 4 Cup Original Flour Blend

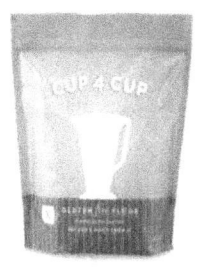

Better Batter Gluten Free Flour

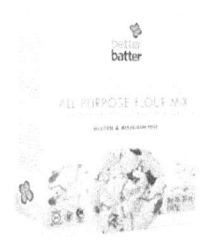

Enjoy Life All-Purpose Flour

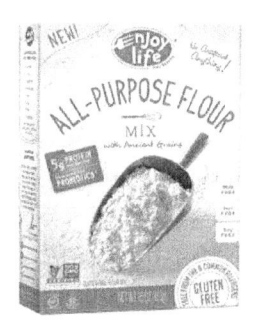

Glutino All Purpose Flour

Gluten-Free Prairie's Simply Wholesome All-Purpose Baking Mix

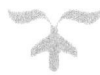

Frozen Meals

7th Annual Gluten-Free Awards:

1st Place: Aldi's LiveGfree Gluten Free Pepperoni Pizza Stuffed

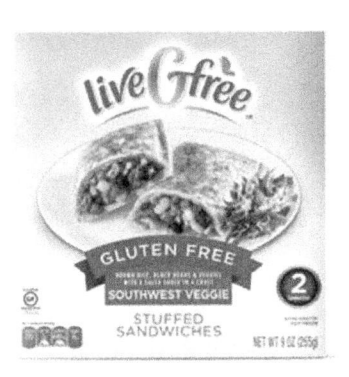

2nd Place: Amy's Kitchen Mushroom Risotto Bowl

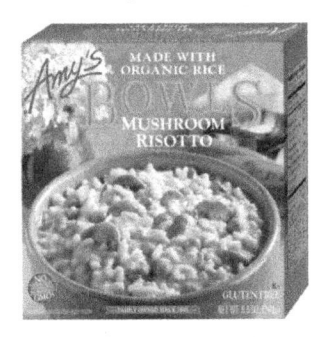

3rd Place: Udi's Broccoli and Kale Lasagna

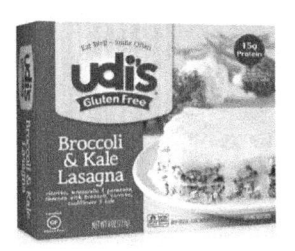

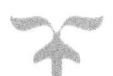

Other nominees:

2017 Gluten Free Buyers Guide

Evol Fire Grilled Steak Bowl

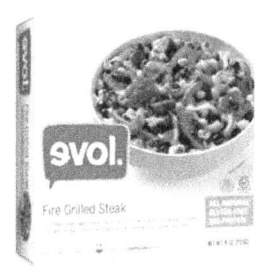

Lean Cuisine Chicken Fried Rice

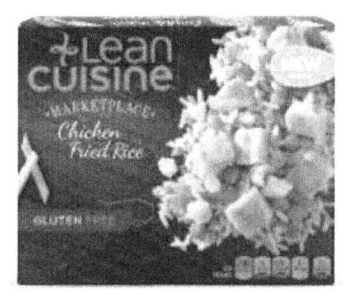

Saffron Road Chicken Pad Thai

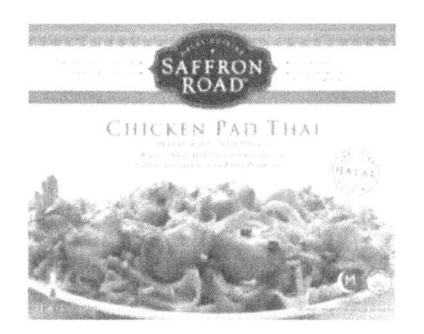

Frozen Pancake & Waffle Brands

7th Annual Gluten-Free Awards:
1st Place: Van's Gluten Free Waffles

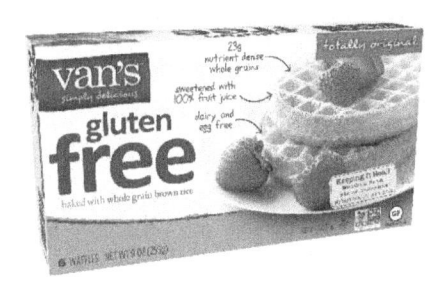

2nd Place: Trader Joe's Gluten-Free Waffles

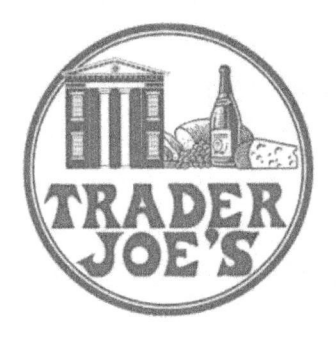

3rd Place: Nature's Path Homestyle Frozen Waffle

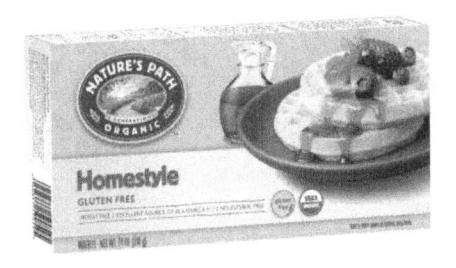

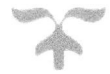

Other Nominees:

Kashi Gluten Free Waffles

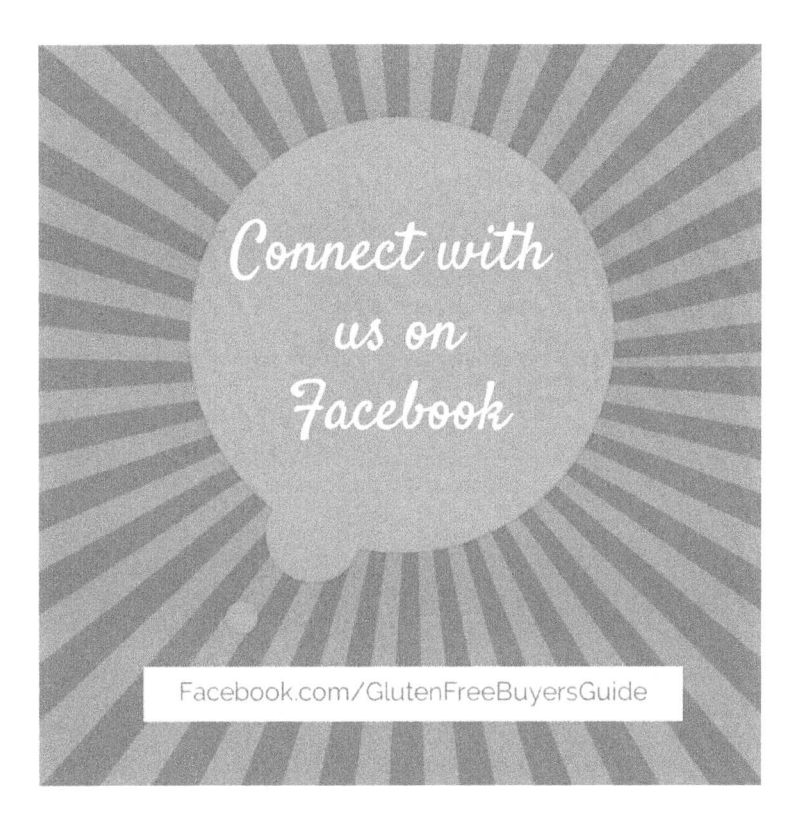

Frozen Pizza Brands

7th Annual Gluten-Free Awards:
1st Place: Udi's

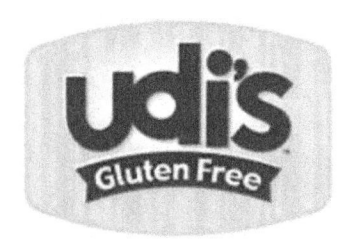

2nd Place: Freshetta

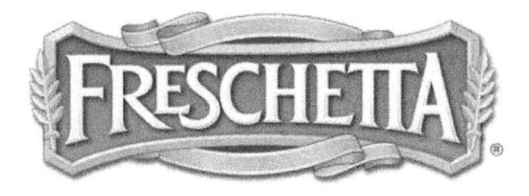

3rd Place: Against The Grain

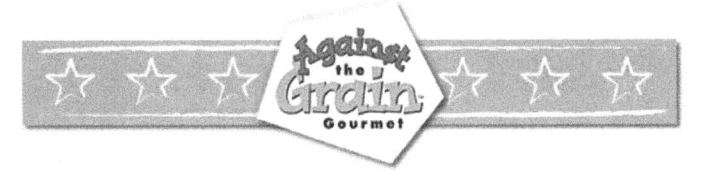

Other nominees:

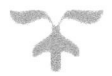

2017 Gluten Free Buyers Guide

Aldi's LiveGfree

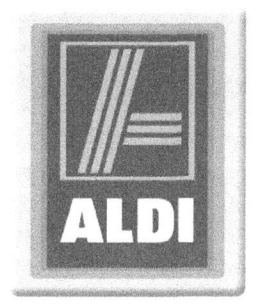

Daiya

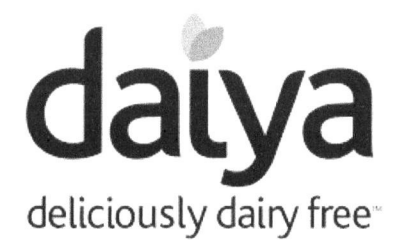

Glutino

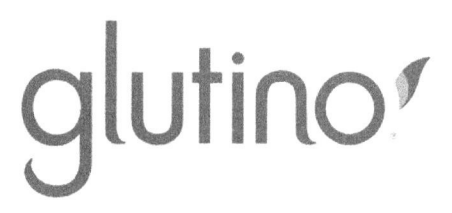

Three Bakers

California Food Company

BOLD Organics

Bella Monica

Russo's

Granola

7th Annual Gluten-Free Awards:

1st Place: Aldi's LiveGfree Gluten Free Double Chocolate Granola

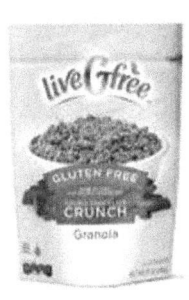

2nd Place: Bakery On Main's Nutty Cranberry Maple Granola

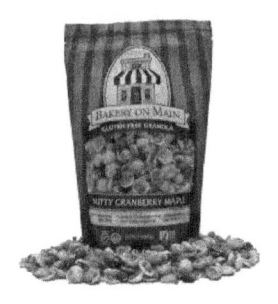

3rd Place: Bakery On Main's Rainforest Banana Nut Granola

2017 Gluten Free Buyers Guide

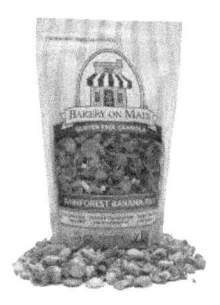

Other nominees:

Purely Elizabeth Original Grain-Free Granola

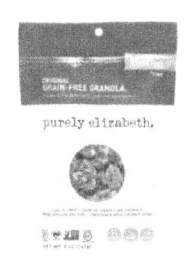

Copia Cranberry Cashew Granola

Jerky

7th Annual Gluten-Free Awards:

1st Place: Oberto Original Beef Jerky

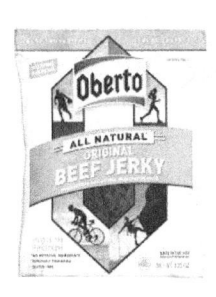

2nd Place: Krave Sweet Chipotle Beef Jerky

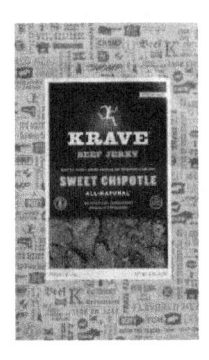

3rd Place: EPIC Bison and Bacon Bites

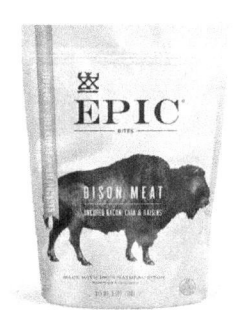

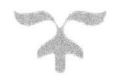

Other nominees:

2017 Gluten Free Buyers Guide

Krave Pineapple Orange Beef Jerky

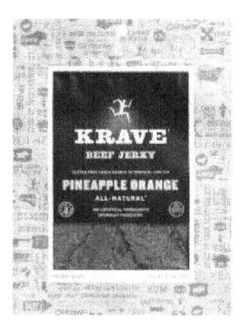

Oberto Spicy Sweet Beef Jerky

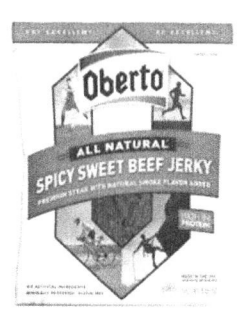

EPIC Cranberry Sriracha Beef Bites

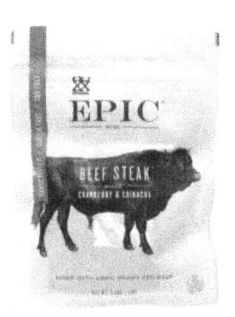

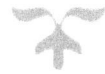

Magazines

7th Annual Gluten-Free Awards:
1st Place: Gluten-Free Living

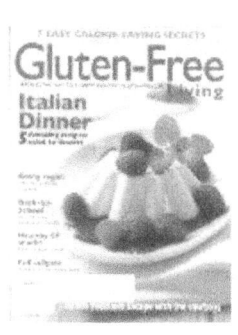

2nd Place: Living Without's Gluten Free & More

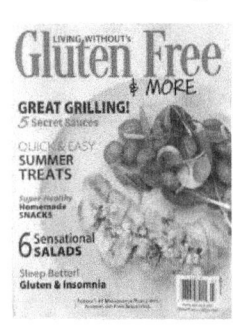

3rd Place: Simply Gluten Free

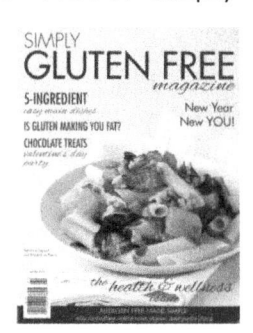

Other nominees:

2017 Gluten Free Buyers Guide

Delight Gluten Free

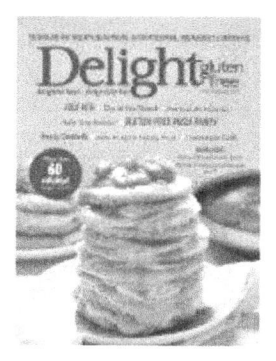

Allergic Living

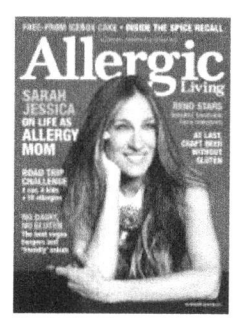

GFF Magazine

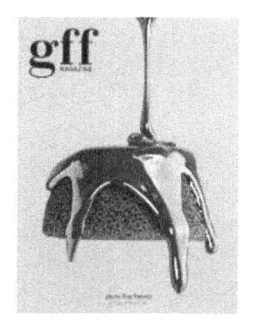

yum.

Mobile Apps

7th Annual Gluten-Free Awards:
1st Place: Find Me Gluten Free

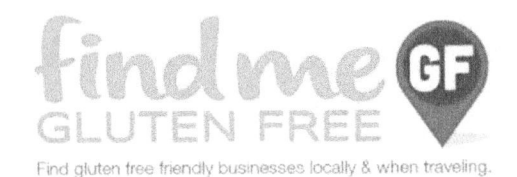

2nd Place: The Gluten Free Scanner

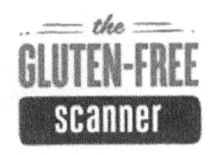

3rd Place: Epicurious

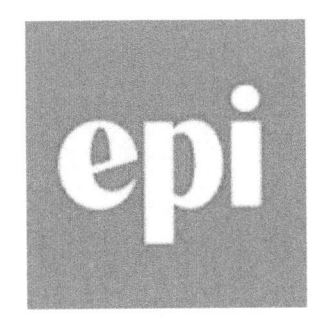

Other nominees:

2017 Gluten Free Buyers Guide

ShopWell

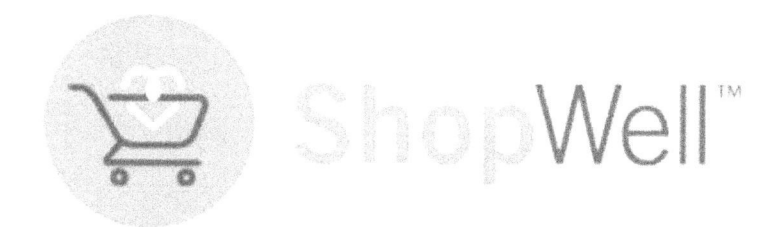

Grain or No Grain

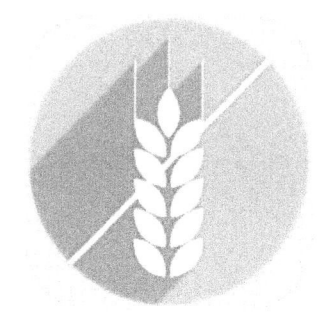

Muffin Mix

7th Annual Gluten-Free Awards:
1st Place: gfJules Muffin Mix

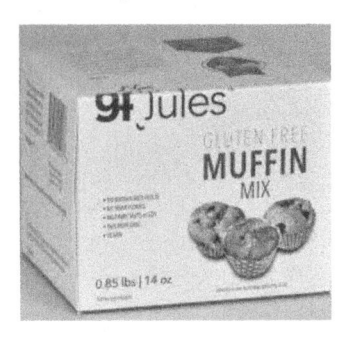

2nd Place: Krusteaz Gluten Free Blueberry Muffin Mix

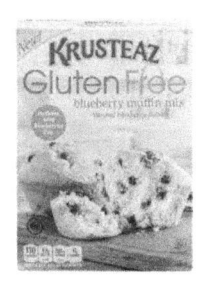

3rd Place: Trader Joe's Pumpkin Bread and Muffin Mix

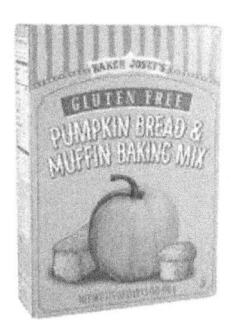

2017 Gluten Free Buyers Guide

Other nominees:

Enjoy Life Muffin Mix

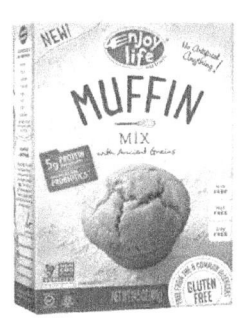

Martha White Gluten Free Chocolate Chocolate Chip Muffin Mix

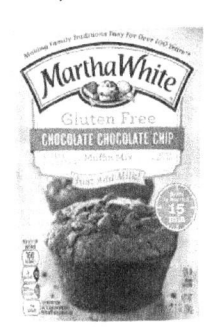

Simple Mills Gluten Free Pumpkin Muffin Mix

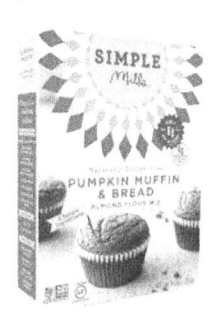

Munchies

7th Annual Gluten-Free Awards:
1st Place: Snyder's Gluten-Free Honey Mustard & Onion Sticks

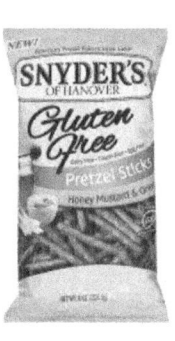

2nd Place: Pirate's Booty Aged White Cheddar

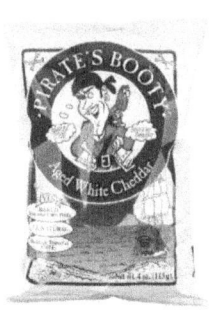

3rd Place: Glutino Buffalo Style Pretzels

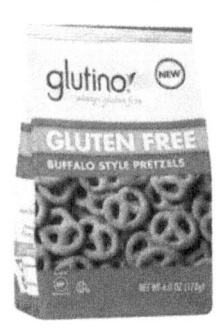

Other nominees:

2017 Gluten Free Buyers Guide

Enjoy Life Ricemilk Crunch Chocolate Bar

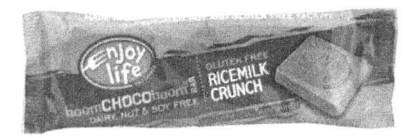

Enjoy Life Garlic & Parmesan Pelentils

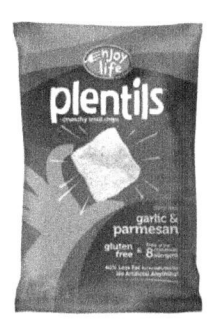

Enjoy Life Mountain Mambo Seed and Fruit Mix

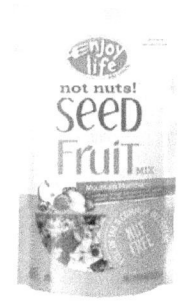

Saffron Road Sea Salt Crunchy Chickpeas (organic)

Beanfields Ranch Bean and Rice Chips

National Restaurant Chains

7th Annual Gluten-Free Awards:

1st Place: P.F. Changs

2nd Place: Red Robin

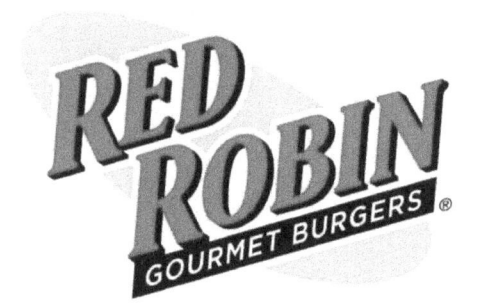

3rd Place: Chipotle

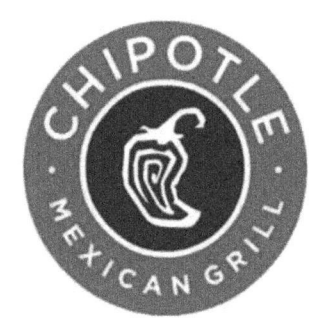

Other nominees:

Outback Steakhouse

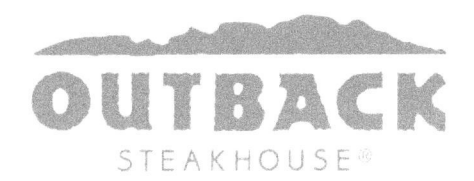

Bonefish Grill

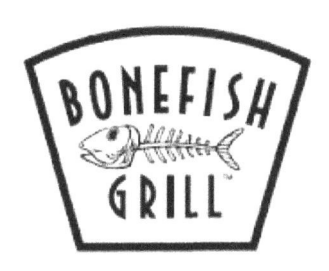

New Products

7th Annual Gluten-Free Awards:

1st Place: Three Bakers Honey Graham Snackers

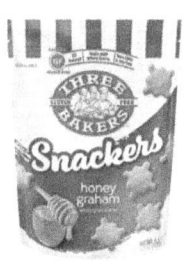

2nd Place: Nima Sensor - Portable Gluten Free Tester

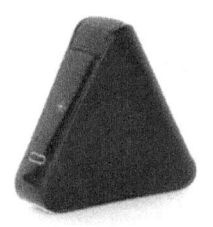

3rd Place: Saffron Road Vegetable Pad Thai

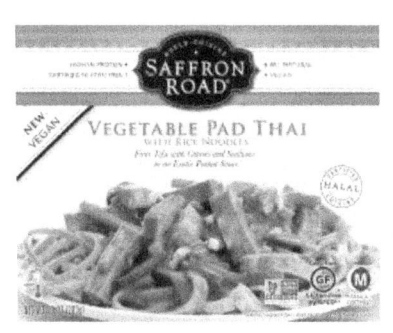

Other nominees:

2017 Gluten Free Buyers Guide

Inspired by Happiness Dreamin' of Strawberries White Chocolate Shortcake

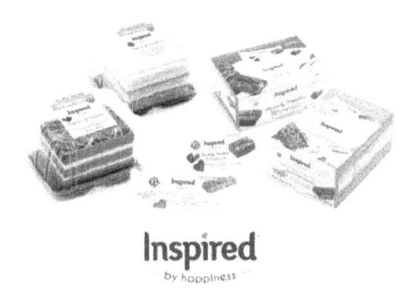

American Gluten Free Subscription Box

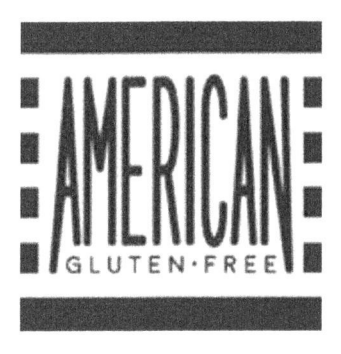

SweetLeaf Stevia Sweetener - Strawberry Kiwi Water Drops

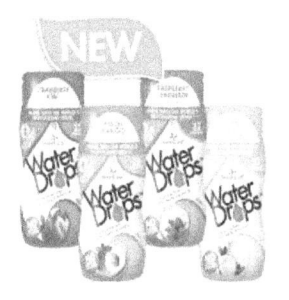

Non-Profits

7th Annual Gluten-Free Awards:
1st Place: Celiac Disease Foundation (CDF)

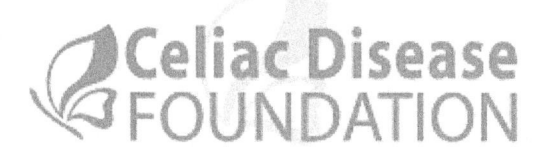

2nd Place: Gluten Intolerance Group of North America (GIG)

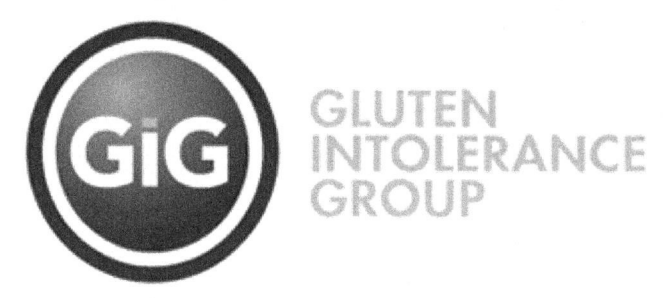

3rd Place: Beyond Celiac

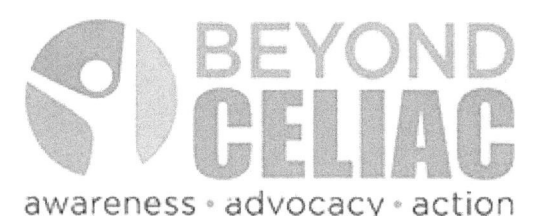

Other nominees:

2017 Gluten Free Buyers Guide

Celiac Support Association (CSA) (formerly Celiac Sprue Association)

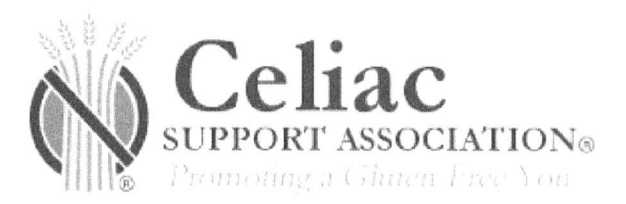

Celiac
SUPPORT ASSOCIATION®
Promoting a Gluten Free You

National Celiac Disease Society (NCDS)

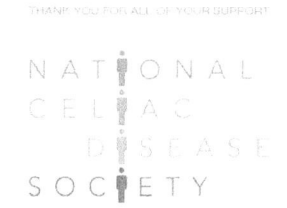

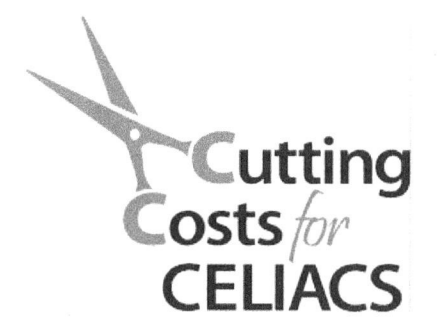

THANK YOU FOR ALL OF YOUR SUPPORT

NATIONAL
CELIAC
DISEASE
SOCIETY

Cutting Costs for Celiacs

Cutting Costs *for* CELIACS

Online Resources

7th Annual Gluten-Free Awards:

1st Place: Celiac.org

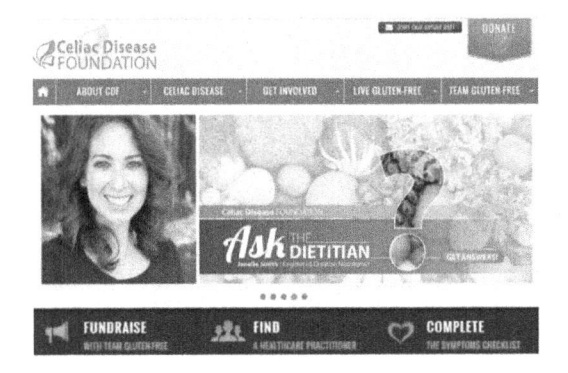

2nd Place: Celiac.com

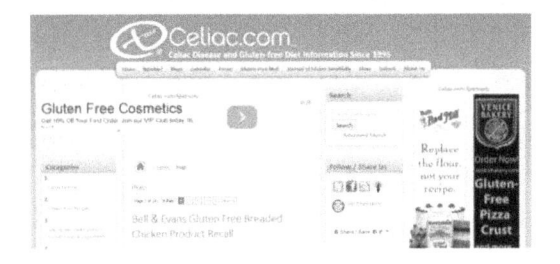

3rd Place: GlutenFreeWatchDog.org

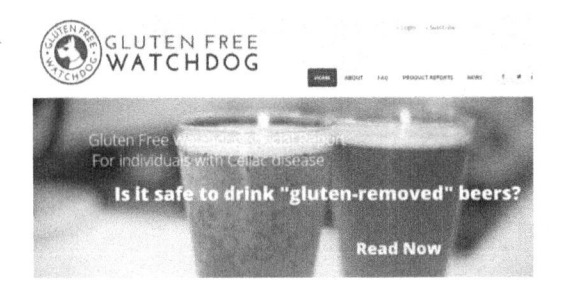

Other nominees:

2017 Gluten Free Buyers Guide

GlutenAway.com

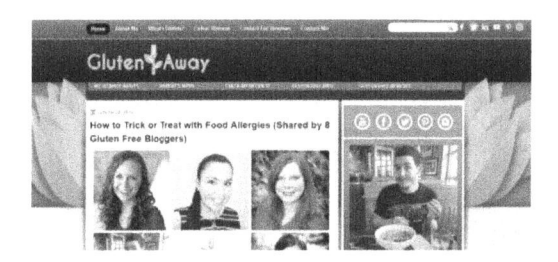

Gluten.org

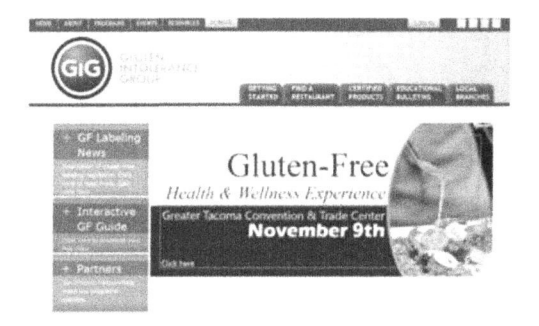

CeliacCentral.org

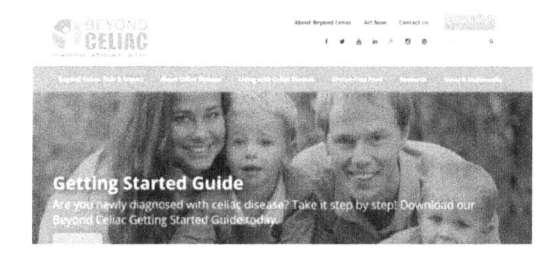

Online Stores

7th Annual Gluten-Free Awards:

1st Place: Amazon

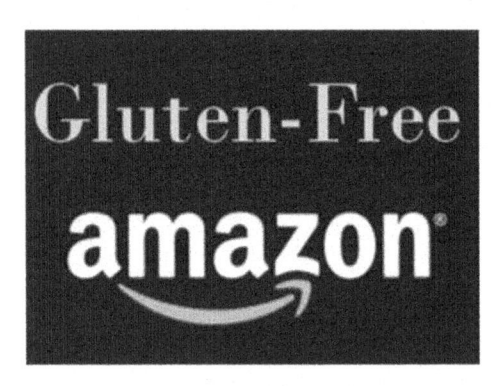

2nd Place: Gluten Free Mall

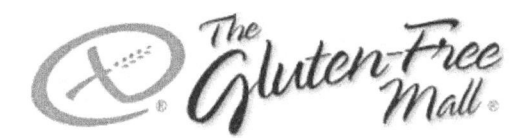

3rd Place: Nuts.com

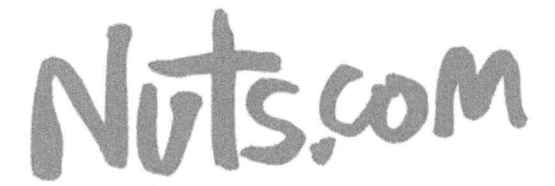

Other Nominees:

Walmart Online

Target Online

Jet.com

2017 Gluten Free Buyers Guide

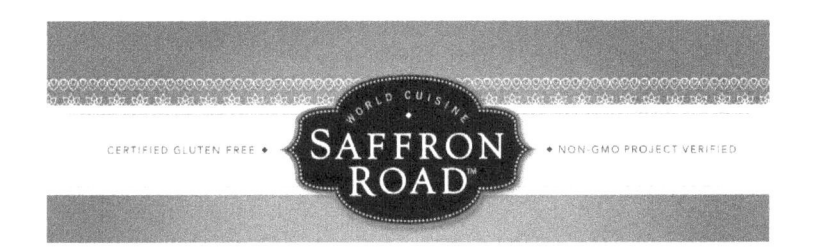

SAFFRON ROAD
World Cuisine

CERTIFIED GLUTEN FREE ♦ NON-GMO PROJECT VERIFIED

Certified Gluten Free Snacks & Simmer Sauces

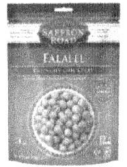

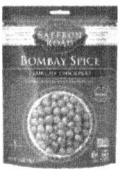

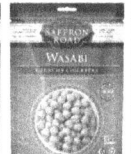

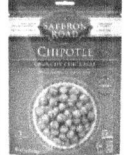

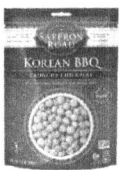

Certified GF Gluten-Free

--- NUTRITIOUSLY ORGANIC CRUNCHY CHICKPEAS ---

Falafel | Bombay Spice | Wasabi | Chipotle | Korean BBQ

--- WORLD CUISINE MEALS IN MINUTES ---

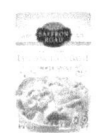

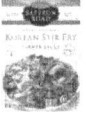

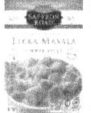

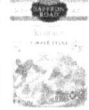

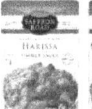

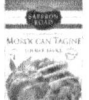

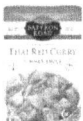

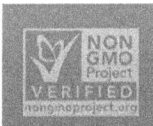

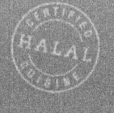

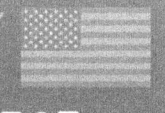

Korean Stir Fry | Tikka Masala | Harissa | Moroccan Tagine | Thai Red Curry

NON GMO Project VERIFIED — nongmoproject.org | Certified GF Gluten-Free | CERTIFIED HALAL CUISINE | PROUDLY MADE IN THE USA

SAFFRONROADFOOD.COM | FOLLOW US ON

Pancake and Waffle Mixes

7th Annual Gluten-Free Awards:
1st Place: gfJules Pancake and Waffle Mix

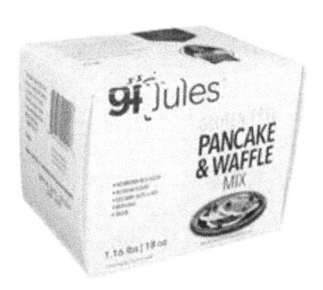

2nd Place: Betty Crocker Gluten-Free Pancake Mix

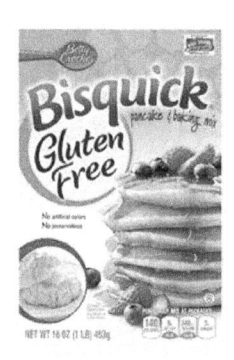

3rd Place: Aldi's liveGfree Gluten Free Baking Mix

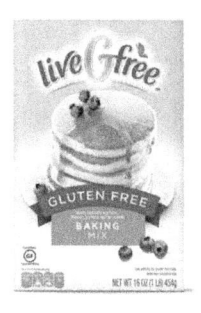

Other nominees:

2017 Gluten Free Buyers Guide

Enjoy Life Pancake + Waffle Mix

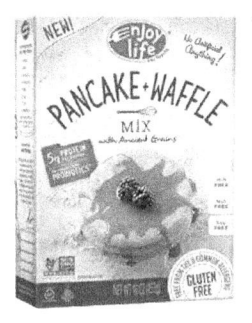

Simple Mills Pancake & Waffle Mix

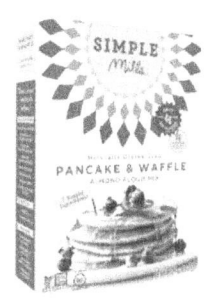

Our House Pancake & Waffle Mix

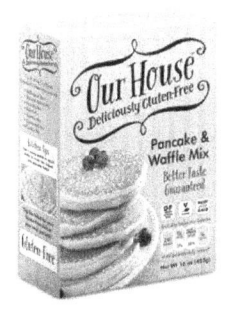

Pastas

7th Annual Gluten-Free Awards:
1st Place: Barilla

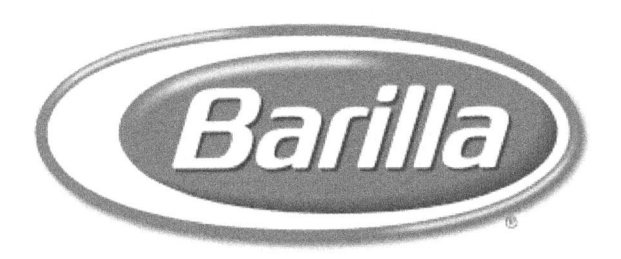

2nd Place: Tinkyada

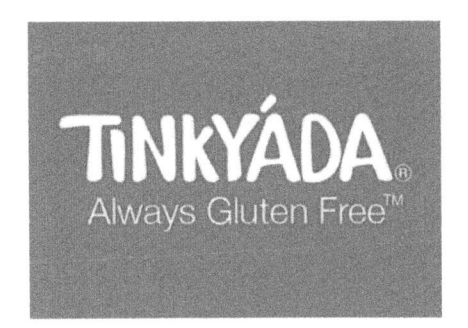

3rd Place: Ronzoni

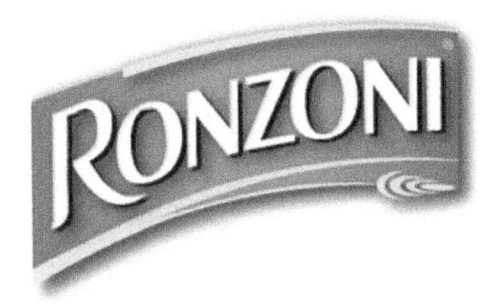

Other nominees:

Quinoa Ancient Harvest

Schar

Jovial

De Boles

Hodgson Mill

Bionature

Heartland

Capello's

Sam Mills

Van's

Explore Asian

Anna

Hannah's Healthy Bakery

Pie Crust

7th Annual Gluten-Free Awards:
1st Place: gfJules All-Purpose Gluten Free Flour

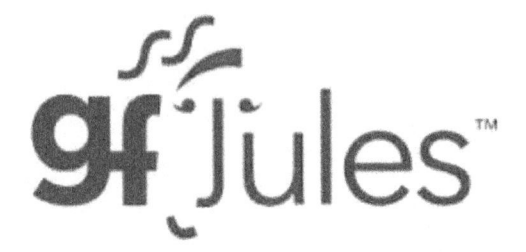

2nd Place: Bobs Red Mill Gluten Free Pie Crust

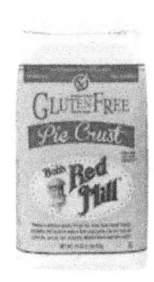

3rd Place: Abundant Love Gluten Free Pie Crust

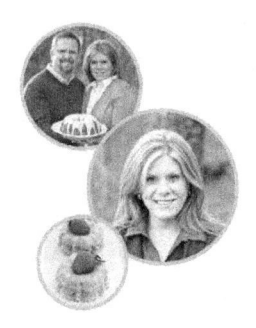

Other nominees:

2017 Gluten Free Buyers Guide 93

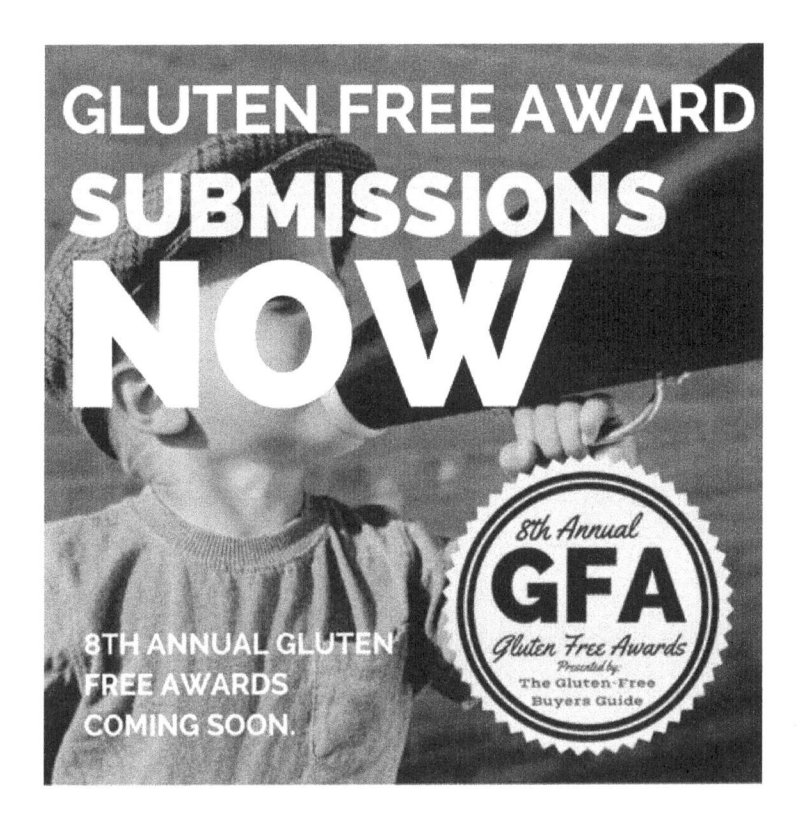

GLUTEN FREE AWARD SUBMISSIONS NOW

8TH ANNUAL GLUTEN FREE AWARDS COMING SOON.

8th Annual
GFA
Gluten Free Awards
Presented by:
The Gluten-Free
Buyers Guide

Pizza Crust Mix

7th Annual Gluten-Free Awards:
1st Place: gfJules Pizza Crust Mix

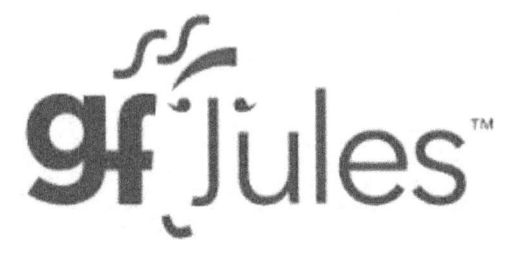

2nd Place: Aldi's LiveGfree Gluten Free Pizza Crust Mix

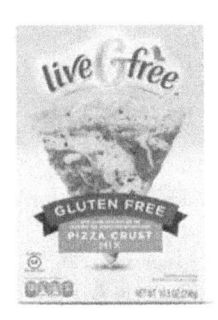

3rd Place: Enjoy Life Pizza Crust Mix

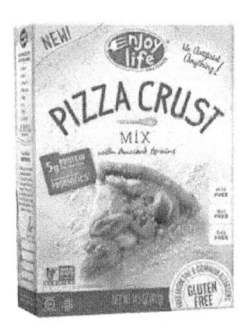

2017 Gluten Free Buyers Guide

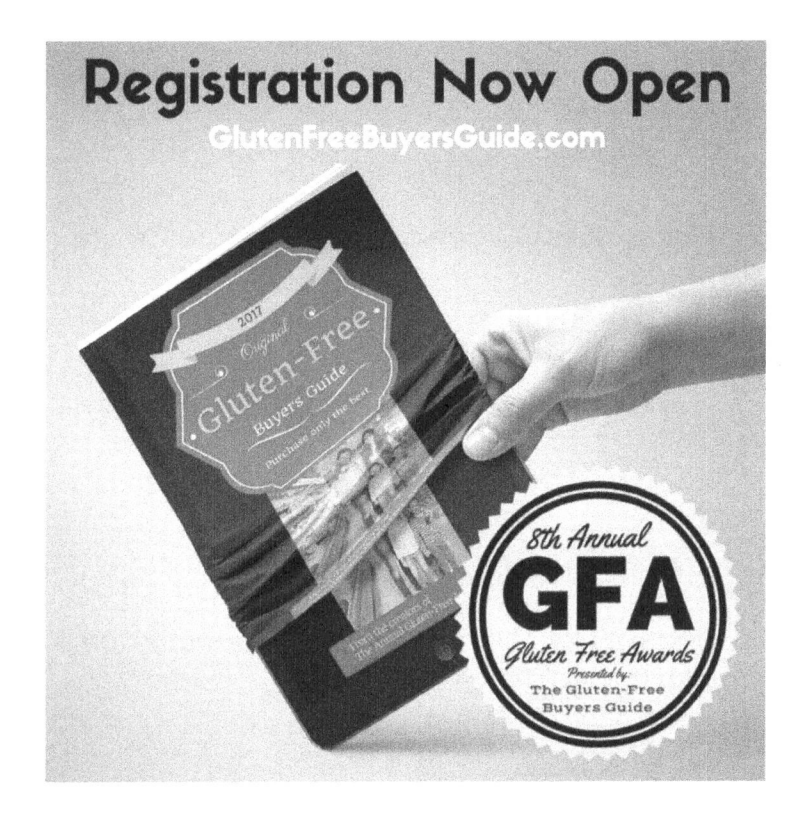

Ready Made Desserts

7th Annual Gluten-Free Awards:
1st Place: Trader Joe's Cupcakes with Buttercream Frosting

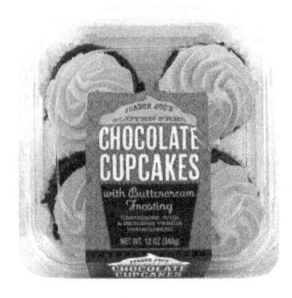

2nd Place: Julie's Organic Gluten Free Ice Cream Sandwiches

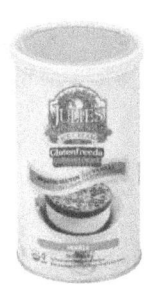

3rd Place: Enjoy Life boom CHOCO boom Ricemilk Crunch Chocolate

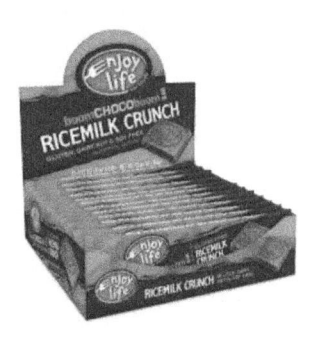

2017 Gluten Free Buyers Guide

Other nominees:

Inspired by Happiness Dreamin' of Chocolate Dark & White Layer Cake

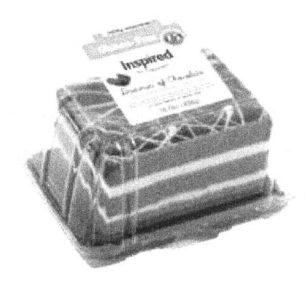

Gluten Free Territory Raspberry Brownies

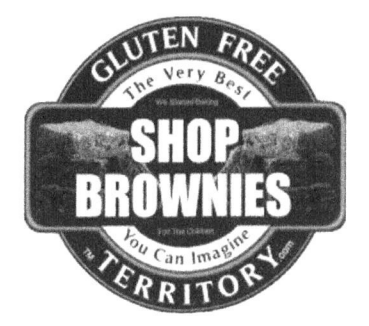

Sauces

7th Annual Gluten-Free Awards:

1st Place: San-J Organic Gluten Free Tamari Soy Sauce (Gold Label)

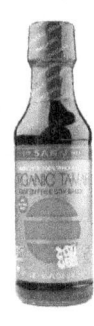

2nd Place: San-J Gluten Free Teriyaki Stir Fry and Marinade

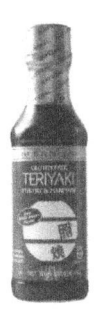

3rd Place: Saffron Road Tikka Masala Simmer Sauce

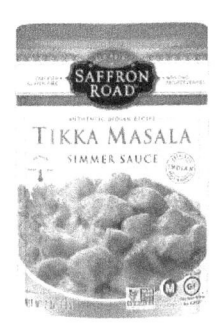

Other nominees:

Saffron Road Harissa Sauce

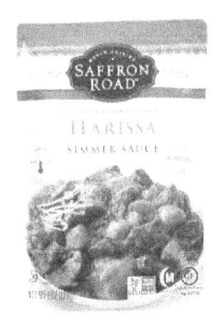

Shopping Guide

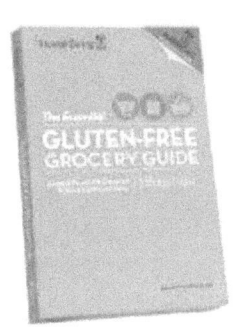

7th Annual Gluten-Free Awards:
1st Place: The Gluten Free Buyers Guide

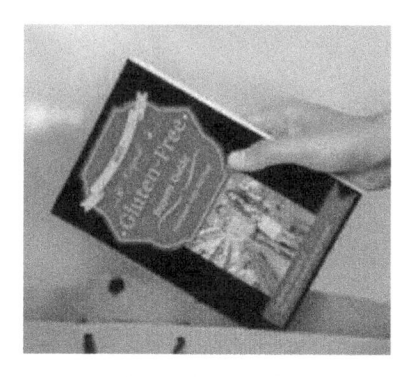

2nd Place: Triumph Dinning

The Gluten-Free Awards
Presented by The Gluten-Free Buyers Guide

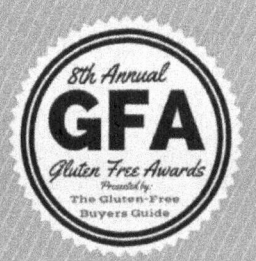

8th Annual GFA — Gluten Free Awards
Presented by: The Gluten-Free Buyers Guide

- 50+ Categories
- Consumer Driven
- Published in Buyers Guide
- Helps New Shoppers
- Helps Category Managers

August 31st: Submissions Due
October 1st: Voting Starts
December: Results Announced

TheGlutenFreeAwards.com

Snack Bars

7th Annual Gluten-Free Awards:
1st Place: Kind Bar Almond and Apricot

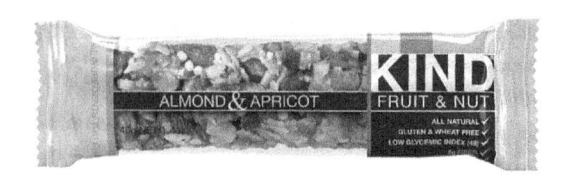

2nd Place: Lara Bar Peanut Butter Cookie

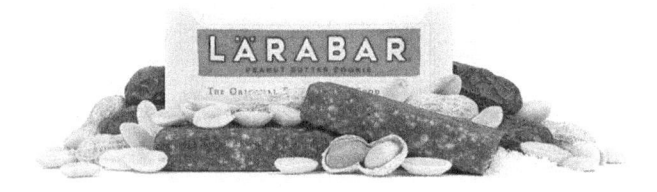

3rd Place: Enjoy Life Cocoa Loco

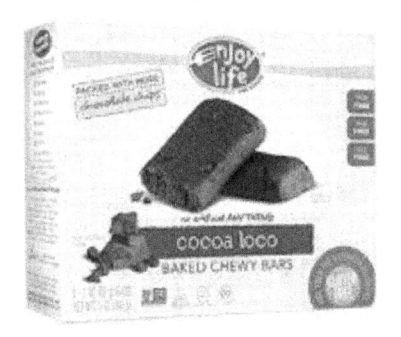

Other nominees:

Aldi's LiveGfree Gluten Free Baked Very Berry Chewy Bars

2017 Gluten Free Buyers Guide

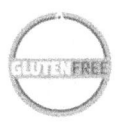

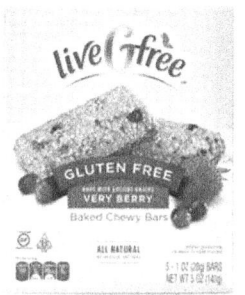

Bakery On Main's 4-4-8 Bars

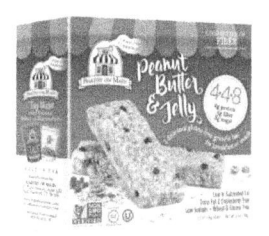

Oatmega Bars

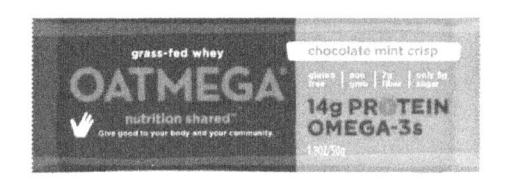

Social Media Platforms

7th Annual Gluten-Free Awards:
1st Place: Facebook

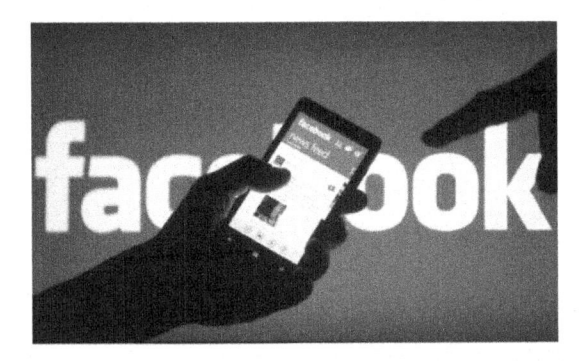

2nd Place: Pinterest

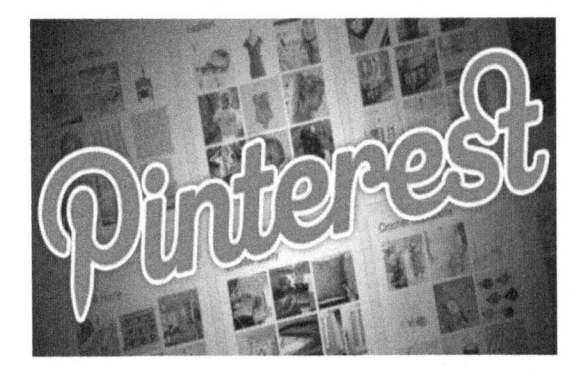

3rd Place: Instagram

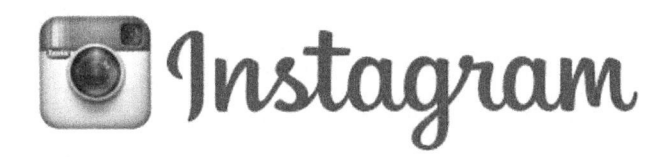

Other nominees:

Gluten-Free Faces

Twitter

Google +

Linked In

Meet-Up

Periscope

Summer Camps

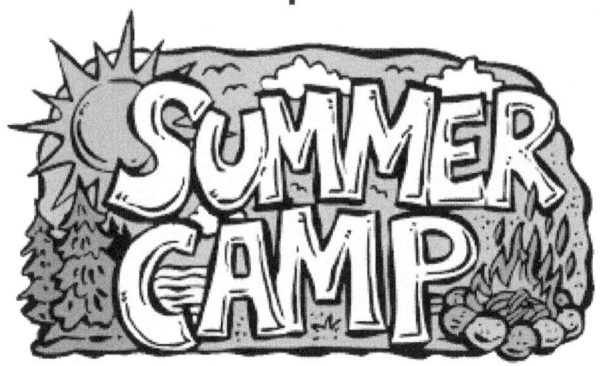

7th Annual Gluten-Free Awards:
1st Place: Gluten-Free Fun Camp Maple Lake, Minnesota

2nd Place: Camp Celiac Livermore, California

3rd Place: GIG (Gluten Intolerance Group) Kids Camp EastCamp KanataWake Forest, North Carolina

Other Nominees:

CDF Camp Gluten-Free™ Camp Fire Camp NawakwaSan Bernardino Mountains, CA

Gluten-Free Overnight CampMiddleville, Michigan

The Great Gluten Escape at GilmontGilmer, Texas

Camp WeekaneatitWarm Springs, Georgia

Gluten Detectives Camp (Day Camp)Bloomington, Minnesota

GIG Kids Camp WestCamp SealthVashon Island, Washington

Camp Silly-Yak Brigadoon Village Aylesford, Nova Scotia

Appel Farm Arts Camp Elmer, New Jersey

Camp Emerson Hinsdale, Massachusetts

International Sports Training Camp Pocono Mountains, Pennsylvania

Camp Celiac North Scituate, Rhode Island

Timber Lake Camp Shandaken, New York

Camp Eagle Hill Elizaville, New York

Emma Kaufmann Camp Morgantown, West Virginia

Foundation for Children & Youth with Diabetes Camp UTADA West Jordan, Utah

Clear Creek Camp Green's Canyon, Utah (Serves Alpine School District children)

Supplements

7th Annual Gluten-Free Awards:

1st Place: Garden of Life RAW Gluten Free Support

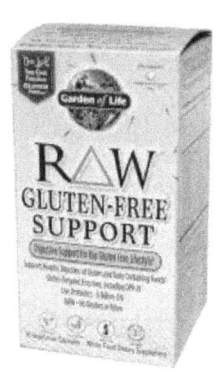

2nd Place: L'il Critters Gummy Vites Multivitamin

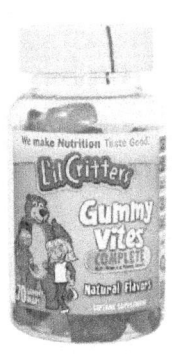

3rd Place: Nature Made Multi

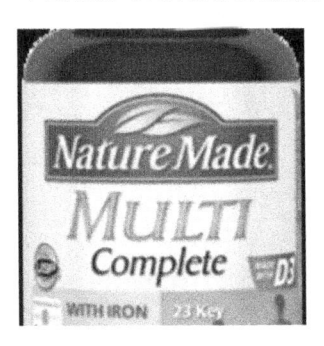

2017 Gluten Free Buyers Guide

Other nominees:

Nordic Naturals Fish Oils

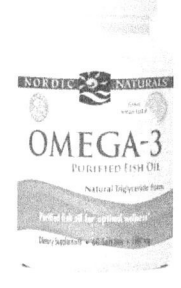

Just Thrive Probiotic

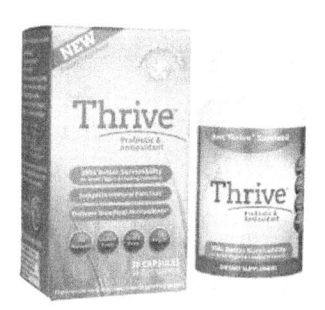

Hyperbiotics PRO-15

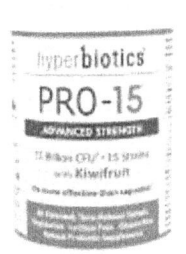

Tortilla or Wrap

7th Annual Gluten-Free Awards:
1st Place: Mission Soft Taco Gluten Free 8ct

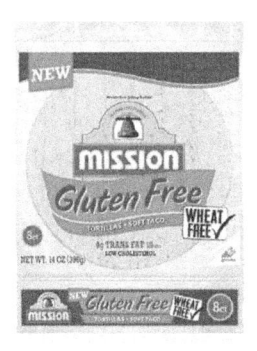

2nd Place: Aldi's liveGfree Gluten Free Plain Wraps

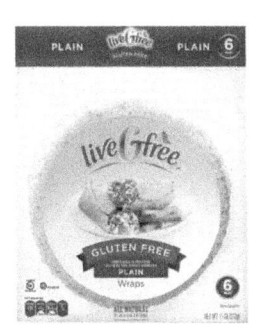

3rd Place: Rudi's Spinach Tortillas

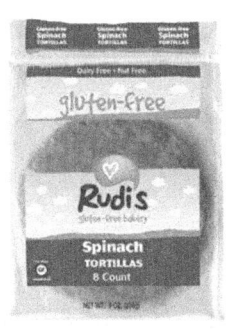

Other Nominees:

Glutenfreeda Sun-dried Tomato & Herbs Gluten-Free Flour Wrap

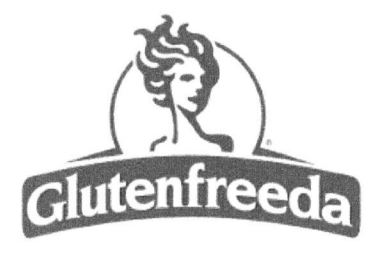

BFree Multigrain Wrap

BFree Sweet Potato Wrap

BFree Quinoa and Chia Seed Wrap

Mi Rancho Organic Corn Taco Sliders

Potapas

Vacation Destinations
7th Annual Gluten-Free Awards:
1st Place: Walt Disney World

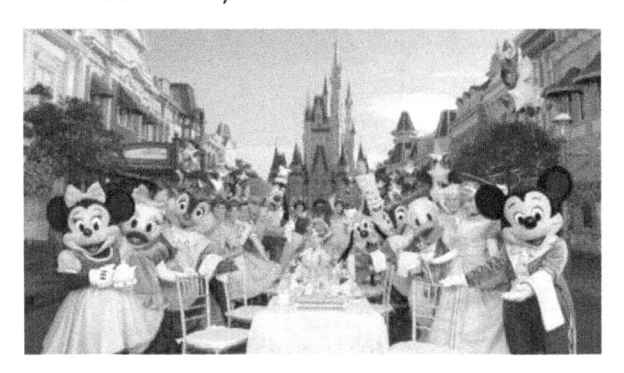

2nd Place: Italy

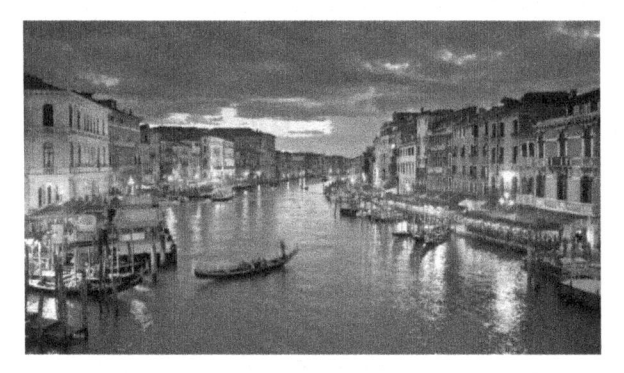

3rd Place: New York City

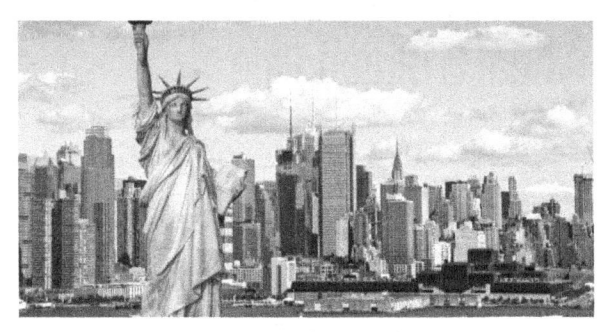

2017 Gluten Free Buyers Guide

Other nominees:

Asheville, NC

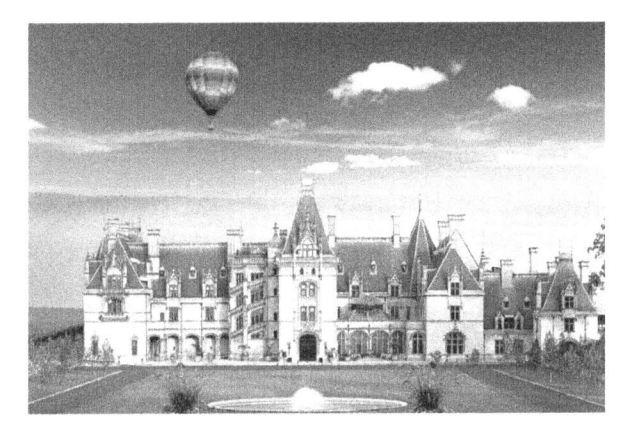

Royal Caribbean Cruises

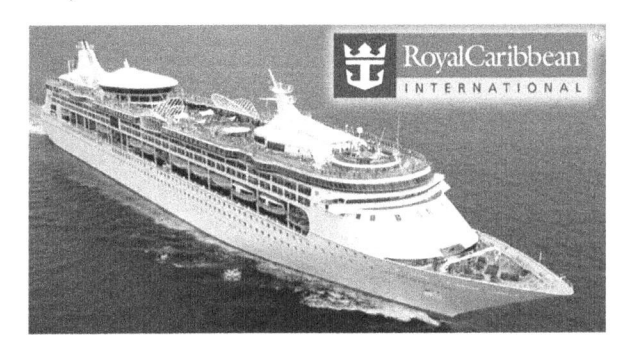

Aulani Disney Resort & Spa in Ko Olina, Hawai'i

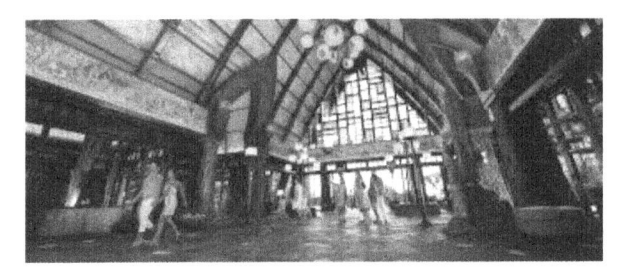

Website

7th Annual Gluten-Free Awards:
1st Place: Gluten Free Watch Dog

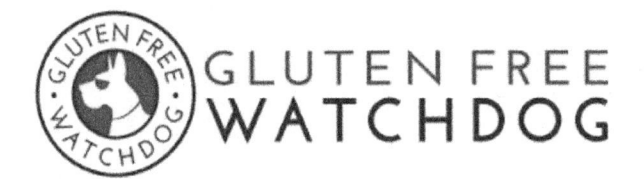

GLUTEN FREE WATCHDOG

2nd Place: Gluten Free Travel Site

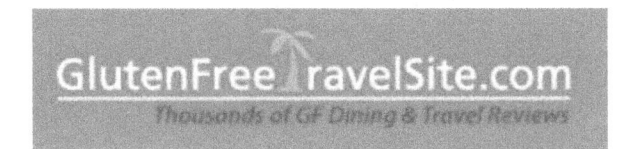

GlutenFreeTravelSite.com
Thousands of GF Dining & Travel Reviews

From our family to yours have a happy and healthy gluten free lifestyle.

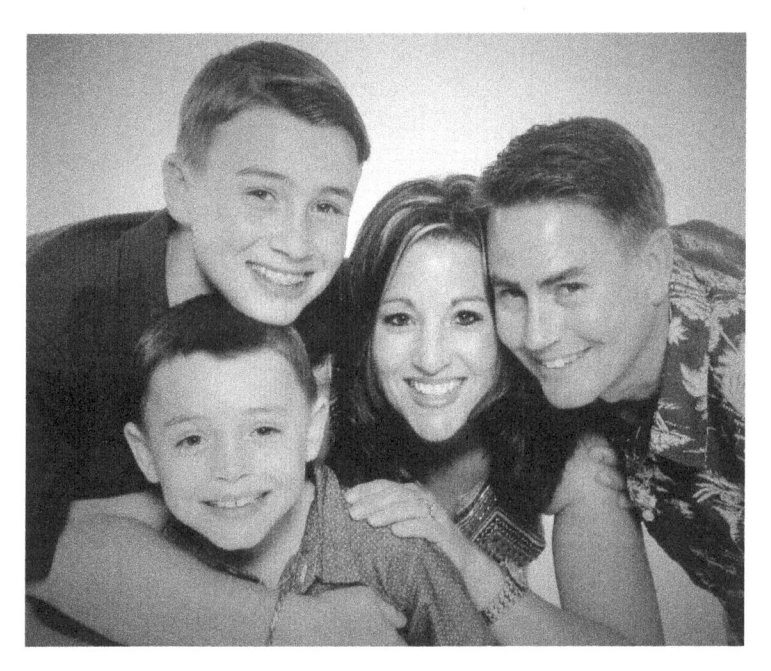

The Schieffer Family

Josh (Dad with Celiac) VP Sales and Marketing

Jayme (Mom) VP Operations

Blake (16) Full time runner and surfer

Jacob (12 Celiac) Full time soccer player

Keep up to date with us, the awards, and future buyer guides at GlutenFreeBuyersGuide.com

Made in the USA
Columbia, SC
13 November 2017